Finding the Doorbell

SEXUAL SATISFACTION
FOR THE LONG HAUL

CINDY PIERCE & EDIE THYS MORGAN

Nomad Press
A division of Nomad Communications
10 9 8 7 6 5 4 3 2 1
Copyright © 2008 by Cindy Pierce and Edie Thys Morgan
The trademark "Nomad Press" and the Nomad Press logo are trademarks of Nomad
Communications, Inc. Printed in Canada.
ISBN: 9780979226854
Questions regarding the ordering of this book should be addressed to Independent
Publishers Group
814 N. Franklin St.
Chicago, IL 60610
www.ipgbook.com

Nomad Press
2456 Christian St.
White River Junction, VT 05001

To my mom, Nancy, for encouraging all seven
of us to follow our hearts and for pulling out the stops
for the Big Questions along the way.
To Bruce, whose bravery and humor bring joy
to every day.
—Cindy

To Nina, who taught me nothing about you
know what, but gave me the key to open my own doors
by showing me that every experience—good, bad,
or horrendous provides great material.
To Chan, for diligently tending to all those
vows, and making it look easy.
—Edie

Contents

Foreword

I t has been five years since I arrived in Paris for my husband's sabbatical. It was not long before I began to notice how openly amorous young Parisians were on the Metro and in cafes, parks, and theatres. I noticed very sexy billboards everywhere, and marveled that advertisers could get away with such salacious displays. There was a soft pornography program on one of the major television stations that aired every single night. Were the French really sexier than Americans, or was a life of leisure distorting my observations?

At the end of my year in Paris, I attended an international conference on female sexual dysfunction. I learned about the conference from a friend who asked that I attend a debate about whether female sexual dysfunction existed as a disease, or was a construct of the pharmaceutical industry. As a healthcare activist who opposed putting profits before patient care, I knew where I stood politically. However, as a woman who had experienced premature menopause as a consequence of high-dose chemotherapy for breast cancer 13 years earlier, I had first-hand experience with female sexual dysfunction.

Dr. Leonore Tiefer was the debater whose side I had been asked to support. Dr. Tiefer is a professor of psychiatry at New York University and the founder of the grassroots organization, A New View of Women's Sexual Problems. It took a lot of courage for her to argue her position in an industry-sponsored debate in front of an industry-sponsored audience at an industry-sponsored conference. After the debate (which she did not lose), she asked me to consider introducing a New View curriculum at Harvard Medical School. It was then I realized there was *no* sexual curriculum at Harvard Medical School. In fact, I realized that I rarely discussed sexual health even with my patients, other than prescribing contraceptives and encouraging safe sex.

Why had I not done more to determine whether my patients were having sexual problems? First, America *is* different from Paris and much of Europe with respect to acceptance of sexuality. Americans are simply uptight about sex. Even those of us who came of age during the sexual revolution in the late 1960s are more repressed than we would like to admit. This repression makes it difficult for patients to ask their physicians about sexual problems, and also makes it uncomfortable for physicians to try to address those problems. Secondly, how can physicians address sexual problems if they don't know much of anything about sex other than their own, possibly rather dreary, sexuality?

Thus, upon my return to Boston and the practice of primary care, I endeavored to introduce sex into the curriculum at Harvard Medical School. A group that included medical students, two anatomists, and clinicians from different disciplines developed a curriculum over one year of meetings and literature research. In the spring of 2005, Human Sexuality in Medicine was offered as an elective for first-year medical students. Nine students signed up, and eight of them were women. The following year, 29 students enrolled, including many men, and 32 attended this past spring. This year, sexual physiology was introduced into the core curriculum for the first time. We are making progress.

After studying human sexuality for three years, I have come to the conclusion that most of us are operating under a set of beliefs and expectations about sex that are either ill-conceived or unrealistic. This ignorance results in considerable personal suffering and relational conflict at some point in most of our lives. While there is diversity in levels of sexual desire, sexual preferences, and activities, there are basic realities experienced by everyone. Sex is necessary for procreation. Sexuality is part of being a living, sentient person. Sex is essential for the health of an intimate relationship. Individual sexuality changes as a function of good and bad experiences, time in a relationship, and aging. Perhaps the most important information I learned and now teach is that men and women need to understand more about each others' sexuality and have open, ongoing communication about their needs.

Cindy Pierce and Edie Thys Morgan have written a wonderful, compassionate, and totally entertaining book about sex in long-term relationships. Readers will be informed about common problems and the solutions that have worked for some couples. Efforts to maintain sexual health must be ongoing and informed by knowledge of how to combat the sexual consequences of stress, aging, and illness. This book will educate and encourage couples to find the compromises necessary to keep sex alive and well throughout their lives together.

Susan E. Bennett
August 12, 2007
Brookline, Massachusetts

Dr. Bennett is 60 years old, married, and the mother of two daughters. She is a primary care physician at Massachusetts General Hospital in Boston, Massachusetts, and an Assistant Professor of Medicine at Harvard Medical School.

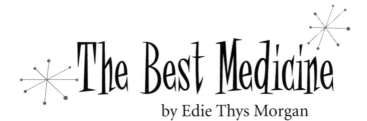

The Best Medicine

by Edie Thys Morgan

Our first research mission for this book took us to our small-town bookstore where, upon leaving, I was relieved that none of our neighbors had seen us camped out in the sex section. As I passed the unusually long line of customers waiting at the register and was eyeing the door and a clean escape, I saw Cindy lean in toward the store manager: "Just thought you should know, the sex section is all out of order," she said softly. "What section?" he answered loudly, in a bid to liven up his morning. "The SEX SECTION!" she yelled, backing away as every head turned to look at us. Outside, she smiled an apology to my red cheeks. "Sorry, but I'm your medicine."

The inspiration for this book came from Cindy's one-woman show, "Finding the Doorbell," in which she describes, among many other intimate details, her first orgasm. The consequence of this event was not only her own sexual awakening, but also, with subsequent investigation, her realization of how few sexually active women were having orgasms on a regular basis. Cindy found this shocking, sad, and nearly criminal. Oh, the missed opportunities! Throughout her life, Cindy has devoted her energies to many things—sports, coaching, teaching, parenting, innkeeping—but her constant underlying mission has been to advocate for "better sex for the people." Not wilder sex or kinkier sex, but the kind of mutually fulfilling sex that brings couples the sense of connection we all crave. Given Cindy's complete lack of stage fright, together with her athletic, theatrical mode of storytelling, a one-woman show seemed the best way to deliver the message.

When it comes to everyday sex banter, Cindy and I are at opposite ends of the spectrum. Whereas she, the youngest of seven, grew up with too much exposure and information, my Puritanical upbringing included exactly zero communication about sex. Despite growing up in free-lovin' California, my vocabulary included "sex" only as it cropped up in the suffixes of distant New England towns. I managed, through two childbirths, to avoid saying the word vagina, ever. This is not to say I did not have or enjoy sex, I just didn't have the tools or the slightest motivation to talk about it. When Cindy met me, she had unwittingly connected with an anonymous yet significant component of her target audience—the Silent Majority.

As our friendship matured, I started saying vagina tentatively in private settings, and when Cindy created her show, it became clear that I could not only be a writing partner but also a barometer for the Silent Majority I represented. As we analyzed feedback from Cindy's adult audience, we realized that many people's open sexual communication stopped after college. Even in good relationships, life goes on, you get busy, and sex is not the top priority. We go into a new relationship expecting that good sex—"good" meaning fulfilling to each partner—will always be there, like a 24-hour mini-mart around the corner. And of course it is, at first. But, if you don't give that mini-mart enough business, the hours get cut back, and eventually the selection dwindles until it's barely worth the detour.

The more Cindy and I talked to people, the more we realized that there was a widespread, unspoken—but nonetheless urgent—desire for a return to full service, or at least some service, in the bedroom. Sex, by itself, may not be something we openly consider a priority, especially as we become overwhelmed by the day-to-day time demands of work, kids, and family. But sex, as it represents an emotional and physical connection, cannot help but be a grounding force in our relationships. It's not like we forget about sex—we are reminded of it on every prime-time TV show and corner newsstand—but we do forget (or are afraid/ashamed) to honor its true value and then it becomes another item on the to-do list. The less we connect in our relationships, the harder it becomes to connect, and hence the spiral into the Silent Majority. As any 40-year-old Puritan knows, talking about sex is awkward. But humor, used judiciously, kindly, and in the spirit of universal cluelessness, is the proverbial spoonful of sugar. It can defuse tension in a charged area of many relationships and ease the communication that fosters more fulfilling sex lives.

The anecdotes in this book are culled from interviews with adults of all ages and both genders; from deer-in-the-headlights college freshmen embarking on their sexual voyage to Alpha-male singles under pressure to "know what women want." From weary parents who struggle to recapture their mojo to experienced retirees who have shed their inhibitions, as well as people who wrestle with the age-old questions like how much sex is normal, and what *really* constitutes good sex.

In taking the covers off other people's intimate experiences we offer perspective on what is normal but also provide practical advice and guidance to a simpler and better sex life. Exhaustive sex info is out there—graphically, mind you, in books, on TV, and on the Internet—but most of us are not getting it. Why? "Great sex" books overstep the sexual expectations most people have, with pictures of people who look like they are trying to devour each other, and advice about toys, porn, and gizmos. Most working parents don't have the time or secure storage for such accessories, let alone the motivation to study an encyclopedia on a natural act that can be done by teenagers in the back of a car. Frankly, three-hour orgasms, 365 positions a year, and driving your man or woman wild is a proposition so daunting as to be a buzz-kill. We do not promise scientific "proof" of any of our theories, but we do promise, at a minimum, lots of laughs and a chance to learn from others in a comfortable way.

What we all have is a unique montage of sexual knowledge and skills in our personal toolbox. We hope the conversations in this book will unclutter, augment, and reorganize your toolbox. This book features a hands-on, gear-free approach to sex. It's because that's enough in itself or at least a starting point for the more ambitious.

Despite our differences, Cindy and I both spent our youth immersed in sports with uncensored access to the male world, and now share an adult network of wise women and men who talk freely about sex-related issues. We have developed an acute awareness of the positive power and healthy attitude that comes with openness and levity about sex. We're working, raising kids, trying to keep our relationships healthy, and seeking to make sex an important part of our lives without it dominating our identity, time, and brain space. We're a lot like everyone out there, but one of us talks about it, a lot, with everybody, and the other takes good notes.

Section I:
Obstacles to a Healthy
Sex Life

by Cindy Pierce

When kids ask, "Why is that book called *Finding the Doorbell?*" adults squirm. It also allows an opportunity to articulate the deeper meaning of the title to those kids and their cringing parents. Finding the Doorbell—in this book and in my one-woman show of the same name—represents the actual sexual awakening of finding and "ringing" the clitoris, an event that occurred for me relatively late in life, in a college library bathroom stall by myself and by mistake. In a broader sense—and this is what you can tell your kids when they see the book on your bedside table—Finding the Doorbell is a figurative process. It represents your power to find happiness by adapting and evolving as you move through the transitional doors in your life.

A collision of factors led to my career in openly talking about sex on stage and in this book. My parents certainly didn't bring sex up around the dinner table during my childhood, but as the youngest of seven children in a country inn, I was surrounded not only by weekend guests and their adult conversations, but also by my unofficial Wise Women Panel of sisters and sisters-in-law. Their banter included graphic advice and discussions about sex, contraception, birth, and the endless trials and celebrations of the female body. They always found humor in what was potentially shameful, converted sexual mishaps into lessons and laughter, and by their example I learned to do the same.

Growing up a tomboy I had a sort of dual gender citizenship, where my guy friends allowed me full access to the male side of life. I served as a liaison between my boy and girl friends. The guys revealed to me that giving orgasms to girls seemed to be a bit of a crapshoot. When I finally did discover my "doorbell," I embarked on a mission of encouraging women toward self-discovery while urging men to get comfortable asking for guidance in complicated territory. My task, as I have learned through the years, is endless, because most adults of all ages and levels of sexual experience are desperate for information and guidance. Hence, the show.

The book concept arose during a 5:30 a.m. run with Edie the morning after a performance/Q+A I had done for 30 fraternity brothers and football teammates from Dartmouth College. After I recapped the event to Edie I noted that the questions and concerns of 22-year-old guys were the same that we were hearing from men our own age and older. Edie had one response: "It's time for a book!"

As we embarked on our research, every woman and man to whom we mentioned the book was brimming with stories, perspective, and ideas to contribute. We assured people their contributions would be anonymous, and they are. However, we were surprised that most of them were unconcerned about anonymity and were actually relieved to unburden themselves of unspoken anxieties—it made them feel "normal" about their sex lives.

How does one get to adulthood and marriage and still need advice about sex?

No matter what examples we grew up with, many of us harbor the hope that "happily ever after" is a mythical, foregone conclusion to every love story, and that our one-and-only soulmate will magically escort us down the path through a storybook life. In reality the path is not well-maintained, and each couple must bushwhack its own trail through the oft-traveled yet vexing territory of long-term commitment. "In good times and bad, in sickness and in health" includes birth, parenting, financial issues, in-laws, housekeeping, career stress, and emotional disconnections, as well as changing bodies and sex drives. An endless parade of victories, setbacks, and challenges await the blissful couple that embarks on a life together. Sex—a big part of what got us together in the first place—would seem to be the easy part.

Sadly, sex tends to get overwhelmed by the to-do list, especially as we start a family. The reasons for this are endless, often complicated, and nearly always hard to discuss. Consequently, for many couples, what was once the passion of the relationship becomes its bane. I once heard that when sex is good it takes up 10 percent of the relationship but when it's not good it takes up 90 percent of it. This supports our belief that sex can be a pillar of the relationship without being its central focus, and should never be an obstacle to connecting.

We started our research for the book by emailing friends, who emailed their friends and so on until our network of men and women of all ages spread virally and grew exponentially. We read up on the latest sex research, as well as the groundbreaking historical studies. We interviewed college students, middle-aged couples, and senior citizens about their experiences, what they knew, what they wished they had known, and what they hoped to learn. As our barriers to asking dropped, we got contributions at the grocery store, the post office, the bank, the soccer field—wherever adults gathered. The overwhelming responses from men and women of all ages affirmed that people are universally relieved when they can talk about sex, so we let them.

This book limits its focus to men and women in monogamous, long-term heterosexual relationships, because that is the relationship realm we know. We see our ongoing desire to maintain the health, quality, and balance of our relationships with our partners as a worthy challenge, echoed by most people we read about, see on TV, hear on talk shows, and interact with in our daily lives. If there are some topics that keep coming up, it is because we firmly adhere to the "skillet-to-the-head" theory of learning. Labrador owners and many parents are familiar with this technique, involving the sometimes forceful reminders of key concepts.

This first section is all about obstacles to a healthy sex life—how they got there and why we need to get by them. Most of us enter adulthood with a sexual understanding that is uniquely incomplete. What is good sex? Who are good lovers and why? What makes a relationship "real" or "good?" Without answers to these questions we fill in the gaps with false assumptions that influence our expectations about sex and, most importantly, the lens through which we see ourselves and our partners.

Whether you are looking for ways to increase your odds for sex on any given day or to quench your thirst after months in the sex desert, ideas about how to keep married sex fresh or guide your partner to your hot spots, tips on how to reestablish balance in your relationship or how to give a proper hand job, you will find ideas in this book from many people who are, or have been, in the same boat. This is our panel of wise men and women, and now it is yours.

♀ ♂

"My mother made it clear getting pregnant would be the end of the world and that we shouldn't do anything because if you do much of anything you will get pregnant." —female, age 71

"I had a pretty legit Catholic upbringing—it was clear you don't stick your wiener in a vagina you are not married to, that people die when they masturbate, etc." —male, age 23

Sources: The Good, the Bad and the Unlikely

O ur adult view of sex, however clear or murky, is shaped by early sexual knowledge and expectations. Most of us as sexual seedlings relied on sources of info that were suspect at best, ranging from harmless fiction to helpful hints to scarring overkill. A precious few had sex detail–oriented parents. Some lucky ones had access to dog-eared how-to sex books pilfered from the bookcase. The less-fortunate girls had a brother with a *Hustler* and some derelict friends, while innocent boys were scarred by overzealous Mrs. Robinson characters. The truly unlucky had traumatic exposures or experiences that delayed or discouraged further discovery. Consequently, a great many of us made it through to adulthood with a smattering of sexual knowledge, and not the core curriculum. We know enough to get the job done but not necessarily enough to get it done with any sort of confidence. It's time to put the blame for our ignorance where it belongs—on a time-honored tradition of lousy sources.

ASSUMPTION JUNCTION

Our misconceptions about sex start with two early assumptions: that everyone else knows more about sex than we do and that sex and love are always neatly intertwined. In truth, a well-informed sex education is more the exception than the rule, and as we all eventually discover, love and sex complicate as well as complement each other. That's the part of the equation that keeps sex from being taught in a purely methodical, rational way. Instead of marching along a linear path toward a clear understanding of sex—as we did with other topics like sports or spelling or driving—most of us were served up knowledge on a need-to-know basis and accrued experience in random spurts. We fortified each morsel of true enlightenment with a new batch of assumptions so that by the time we figured out that your hands will not sprout hair or grow warts if you touch yourself, that you don't actually get a girl pregnant from making out, and that the act of sex does not involve either party peeing into or onto the other, the only thing we trusted was our own ignorance.

Instead of starting out our sexual lives with healthy curiosity we start ashamed—either of our inexperience or of our appallingly inappropriate/embarrassing experience. At the core of this shame is the assumption that everyone else "got the memo" and has moved happily and actively along the sexual-mastery continuum. Whatever the cause, shame isn't conducive to healthy communication about sex.

GUILT

Most people's recollections about early sexual thoughts and experiences share one universal theme: Guilt. One 52-year-old woman recalls the extreme circumstances that created her perfect storm of guilt. The only daughter in a large, devoutly Catholic family, she was working on a cruise ship many years earlier and fell for a randy British coworker who led her down the path to multi-orgasmic sex (19 in one night but who's counting). She was having sex with full abandon for the first time in her life. A fire in the engine room caused the ship to go down in the middle of the night and she found herself adrift in the ocean in a lifeboat full of panicked fellow passengers for three days in nothing but her nightie without underwear. "The whole time on that lifeboat I was convinced that God sank the ship because of all that great sex I was having."

> "I always knew that sex was BAD!! I knew my mother would be so disappointed in me that I wouldn't be able to face her. That is why I waited until I was 18, which at the time seemed so old."
> —female, age 32

PARENTAL INPUT, OR LACK THEREOF

Today, pro-active parents are advised to have "the talk" in first grade, age-appropriate educational picture books abound, and toddlers shout, "Mommy my vagina itches" in the middle of Kmart. This is a relatively new phenomenon. In our research, we were primarily interested in where people obtained their early sex knowledge. We were amazed at how, almost universally, parents seem to have been a poor resource for sexual information. Most of us grew up with very little open talk about the land down under. Being left in the dark is a tradition recounted repeatedly by people of all ages. The parental advice that did occur seems, too often, to have consisted of scare tactics.

Cautionary advice was plentiful . . .
- don't give your milk away for free
- don't start doing it because then you'll be expected to do it all the time
- a hard-on has no conscience
- don't have sex until you are married

. . . but nothing that would truly inform. Parents who came of age in the '60s and '70s seem to want to offer more wisdom, but remarkably few had the ability to talk freely and coherently about sex. Rather than hypocritically preach abstinence, many shoved "educational" material at their kids and told them to "just read it and come to me with any questions." Those materials ranged from the instructions on a box of tampons and pads, to the substantially more thorough *Where Did I Come From?* by Peter Mayle. Legions of girls depended on Judy Blume's *Are You There God, It's Me Margaret*, to fill the information void.

> "Judy Blume's book was the only sex ed I had. When I was in fourth grade I said, 'Mom, why do male and female turkeys have breasts?' and she said 'You need to ask your sister about anything to do with that.' That was it. She didn't even answer about turkeys. So that book was a godsend because until I read it I thought when a woman got her period she had to lie on a bench and put a tampon on her stomach while the cramps went away."
> —female, age 42

Many boys didn't even have the pretext of menstruation or the threat of potential pregnancy to initiate a discussion—some were left to educate themselves with the occasional illicit *Playboy* and the barest of clues.

"My Dad came into my room to give me the talk. He'd start to say something then trail off with 'and you know . . .' as if I could fill in the blanks. I was thinking, 'I'm 11! No, I don't know!' Afterward he said, 'I'm glad we had this talk. I was like, 'about what?'"
—male, age 37

Helpful parental sex talk, when it did happen, ranged from the extremely rare, total openness (doctors and veterinarians were notoriously good at this) to the well-meaning and creative parents who employed props like puzzle pieces that fit together, outlet and plug demonstrations, or graphic pop-up books. To their credit, some parents insisted on telling their kids the truth rather than blurring things with tales of storks or cabbage patches.

"I had a conversation with my mom when I was in high school about the slut/stud double standard. My argument was that it wasn't fair that girls get a bad rap, and she shut me down immediately by saying the double standard exists because girls get all the consequences, which of course isn't fair either. I thought my mom was so old-fashioned at the time, and that she really didn't understand. But as an adult, I think I'd tell my own daughter the same thing, although less harshly."
—female, age 32

MORE THAN YOU NEEDED TO KNOW

Ah, you may be thinking—if only my parents had been more open about sex I wouldn't have any hang-ups. Perhaps, but the opposite extreme also has a price, as described by a woman whose free-speaking mother slipped "cunnilingus" into casual conversation when she brought friends to the house. The daughter became so reticent about bringing boyfriends home that her father took her to lunch across from a gay and lesbian bookstore to broach the topic of her sexual orientation. Too much early information can zap the romantic notions of sex.

Involved parents assume the risk of getting more than they bargain for, like the father who allowed his high school–aged daughter to take a college-level course in human sexuality but got concerned on the day porn was to be shown. Dad showed up to monitor the situation and unexpectedly found himself assigned to recount his "first masturbation" for the class. His daughter discovered in horrifying detail what we all know to be true: No matter how old you are, hearing about your parents' sex life is *gross*.

> *"My parents approached sex as something as natural as eating: it involves our bodies, sustains us, entertains us. We had lots of groovy '60s books—with pictures and hand drawings; I also had a cool Swedish doll that was anatomically correct. I can't think of anything my mother didn't tell me. There were times when I'd say, 'OK, enough, I don't want to hear about your orgasms.' Being a bit over-exposed to sexual content . . . actually made me less promiscuous."*
> —female, age 40

Some of us lived our entire youth convinced we were products of the immaculate conception or wondering if our parents still "did it," while others of us discovered it the hard way, in full-color, searing mental images. Most of us could piece together the truth if we dared. One man recalls that every Sunday after church, when his father's work as pastor was done, the door to his parents' bedroom was locked. Another young woman clearly remembers walking to the store with her dad one summer afternoon, then discovering the recently purchased can of whipped cream in her parents' bedroom. The universal gag response to any discovery of, or reference to, our parents' sex lives assures that parents can only tell us so much, and their willingness may drive us further away.

GOOD OLD-FASHIONED SEX-ED

The only real sex education traditions that have passed down through generations are the methods of filling in the gaps. For that, we rely, like those before us, on siblings and friends, camp, scouts, sports teams, the schoolyard, the school bus, merciful neighbors, farm animals, and fortuitous discoveries of all manner of literature from *National Geographic* and Harlequin Romances to *Hustler*. *Penthouse Forum* is fondly remembered as THE go-to resource for males in the '70s, the *Joy of Sex* was a bookcase treasure for curious babysitters, and many enlightened neighborhood moms with a backlog of *Cosmo* and *Ms.* magazines offered more than lemonade.

> *"My Dad gave me the talk. You know—sex is holy, between two people. But the summer before getting to college I felt like I had to have sex before getting to campus."*
> —male, age 21

Despite all that information, many of us had little experiential sharing, and left high school believing we were the Last Virgin Standing. LVS syndrome is still common among men and women entering college and adds to the general anxiety that if you miss the boat on having sex in high school, you are destined to be stranded on your very own virgin island.

College is the Promised Land of sex info, fertile territory for acquiring and sharing both information and actual experiences. These four years of bonding through partying, dating, listening in on roommates, and re-capping all of the above over breakfast at noon does build up a decent bank of knowledge, no matter how much you are actually "getting." College kids are old enough to be having sex out of the shadows and in an environment where they can also talk and learn about it. Some time after we have milked the communal living experience dry, our info sources dwindle—both in numbers and ease of access.

> *"I've always thought the best commencement advice would be along the lines of 'Got any questions? If so ask them now because this global-village-open-exchange thing is about to end forever.'"*
> —female, age 41

Welcome to adulthood. Would someone please turn on the lights?

WHAT DO *WE* KNOW?

Cindy: "My sisters and I asked our mother about sex as a last resort because she wasn't eager to discuss sex openly. Her blowtorch style of launching unsettling wisdom bombs kept us from asking anything for years."

Edie: "I skipped fifth grade. That must have been when it all went down because I don't remember getting any formal information at school. Of course, the informal stuff was all over the place."

BOTTOM LINE

We all have gaps in our education and experience that can ultimately get in the way of our relationships. You did not miss the memo, you did not fail the test, and you are in good company.

WHY SHOULD YOU CARE

Understanding that everyone's sexual knowledge is uniquely incomplete takes the pressure off you by keeping your expectations realistic. Relaxing or releasing feelings of guilt or inadequacy boosts your odds for good sex.

WHAT YOU CAN DO

If you don't feel comfortable or confident in your sexual knowledge, we think it's healthier and more constructive to admit it than to fake it. Look back on your education, or lack thereof, identify the missing pieces, and be honest about them with your partner. We'll get to pleasing others later, but as a first step, understand the source of your limitations. With a positive willingness to fill in those gaps, you can turn ignorance into a healthy curiosity and a good source of humor.

♀ ♂

"I finally told my husband in so many words 'Look pal, my women friends save your ass on a regular basis. When I am ready to kill you, they listen (well) and also point out your good points. You should be sending me out regularly!'"
—female, age 35

"I used to share all kinds of stuff with close friends, mostly college buddies. But that changed once we all were married. It's one thing to share a story about a not-too-serious girlfriend, it's another to share a story about your lifelong partner."
—male, age 41

Tribes and Tools

As we age, theoretically mature, and turn our attention toward building career and/or family, there is less time to devote to niggling questions about sex that we feel we ought to know anyway. Our knowledge consists of whatever we have managed to assemble in our own toolboxes as well as the upgrades and insights that are offered to us by our partners. The open forum of sex banter that many of us experienced during college among a wide group of friends and acquaintances of the same gender is an example of what we like to call a "healthy tribe." Other valuable perspectives come from the trusted advisors from various aspects of our lives who become what we refer to as our Panel of Wise Women or Men. These tribes and panels are often replaced by a more isolated existence and the pressure to "just know it" when it comes to matters of sex and life in general. Furthermore, when we are with a life partner we feel a duty to honor a more evolved level of intimacy by not discussing it outside the relationship.

WHY WE NEED TRIBES AND PANELS

As our relationships mature, and the family unit naturally becomes more insular, paradoxically our need for good sounding boards becomes even more important. It's not realistic or even fair to depend on one person to provide both our most intimate relationship and all the perspective on it. Yet if we don't have regular access to our tribes and panels to remind us of what the baseline for normal is for our gender and age, to act as sounding boards, and to offer advice, we tend to bury, ignore, or silently stew over our questions and concerns. We think that you need both—periodic exposure to the healthy tribe and a comfortable relationship with the panel. We may by default get our information on relationships and sex from "Oprah," the "John Tesh Show," the AP Wire, and other media sources that highlight the latest studies, surveys, and statistics. There's no shame getting what you can out of those messages, but we need to be aware of their limitations and especially how they can unwittingly feed our own pre-existing assumptions. For one thing, the chances of finding your specific concerns addressed in the

> *"I had a lot of sex as a young adult, but I didn't ask questions because I didn't want to be perceived as not knowing what I thought everyone else already knew. Boy, was I wrong. I feel like I missed out on an invaluable experience because of my pride and naiveté. If only I'd had a panel all these years!"*
> —female, age 43

35 minutes you happen to be in the car or folding laundry in front of the TV are pretty slim. When it comes to "facts," statistics can be interpreted in many ways depending on what the researchers are trying to prove and surveys go to a targeted audience that may not share much with you. Even well-done studies may be reported in a way that highlights only the message the writers or TV and radio hosts are trying to promote, ignoring other critical factors. The quest for readership and ratings seems to lead mass media inevitably to display extreme behaviors. If what you see or hear makes you feel inadequate, it's probably because you are, in fact, within the normal range.

ASSEMBLING YOUR PANEL

We suggest that a more satisfying path to understanding the issues that affect your relationship and sex life lies in cultivating and maintaining a panel of wise women and/or wise men who alone or collectively serve as your life raft.

> *"The Coven is the gaggle of women for whom I feel the most connection and affection. They are battery charging, affirming, and offer effortless giving and receiving. I refer to them as the Coven because I sense magic in all of them and they make me feel magical as well. I rarely see the Coven—but they are in my core."*
> —female, age 42

Whatever you call it, these people can be your go-to resource for the information your upbringing or experiences have not delivered.

Friends are the family you choose, and they may develop into many different panels composed of lifelong childhood pals, college buddies, and even entire families seamlessly integrated with each other.

Panel members are much like the sources we had as kids, but upgraded with at least better information and, with luck, empathy. Their wisdom may stem from their deep understanding of you, from their proximity to you in the trenches, or from their willingness to tell it to you straight. A good panel can provide new information but also help you make sense of the information you already have by fielding questions, relating personal experiences, offering ideas, dispensing tough love, and finding humor. They can embolden you, comfort you, encourage you, or even kick you in the butt when necessary.

Panels reward the brave. When you open up the topics of sex and relationships, you run the risk of getting slammed with more details and truths than you may be ready to hear, but the best advice can come from the most unexpected or unlikely sources. The more of yourself you put out there, the more you tend to get back. If you are willing to ask questions and sift through the slurry of uncomfortable, nauseating, or embarrassing stories, you will be rewarded with gold nuggets of relationship-saving perspective.

> *"My group of guys and I talk about all things sexual and scatological, often in combination. We also talk work. We may dive into parental things, but we're not exploring deep, personal feelings and fears. What prevents a more real, sensitive exchange? I think it's cultural. Many guys do not appear to operate on those levels. For those of us who do, exchanges simply aren't made."*
> —male, age 41

MEN AND THEIR TRIBES

Any of you men who have drifted, WAKE UP! This is no time to snooze or skim. Panels are not reserved for women and sensitive, ponytail guys. To be sure, it is far easier for women to find and grow their panels, especially as they mature and are culturally and socially pushed toward each other. From playgroups to bookgroups, women are encouraged and even forced to gather, chat on the sidelines, carpool, and relate. Meanwhile, men often seem to start out with strong social groups in their youth, forging bonds on sports teams, at boarding school, in fraternities, in the military, and under any intense conditions (we find that shared suffering really boosts the openness). But men more often than not abandon their panels after college when our culture discourages them from pursuing or maintaining close male networks. Sex isn't socially acceptable office chatter, and when it comes to deep, thoughtful, and especially sexually based conversation, caveman-like detail is the cultural expectation for men.

One man notes that beyond the occasional off-handed (and usually crude) comment, "we are on our own and up against cultural and social barriers." Few men resort to calling each other "just to talk." The nature of male bonding is summed up in this man's recollection from La Maze class.

"During one class they had the men and women break up into two groups to talk amongst ourselves. When we reconvened and debriefed the women had talked about all kinds of issues and feelings. Meanwhile the guys hadn't said a thing until one of us had the guts to ask, 'Hey, any of you guys gotten laid lately?' So we spent the whole time talking about not getting laid. Guys just want to know that they aren't the only ones suffering." —male, age 40

"My closest friends are the guys I've been playing with (skiing, biking, etc.) for years and years, where there is so much history and common ground that the relationships run deep. My weekly bike race includes a leisurely ride to the course, a race, a leisurely ride back, and then dinner. This event is hard wired into my schedule every Tuesday so my wife, my kids, my colleagues know that if I'm in town, I'm doing the weekly ride." —male, age 43

Whatever it is in our culture that makes men unable to even stop the car and ask for directions has also funneled men toward emotional autonomy. They are expected to be strong, suck it up, and deal with it. However, the men who manage to keep their youthful panels alive, or at least maintain regular exposure to their tribes, are better equipped to weather the inevitable storms that circulate around sex and relationships. The fact that men seem inherently less likely to maintain panels than women (blame it on genetics or society) makes it especially important for men to carve out time in their lives to spend with their healthy

TOOL TIME FOR THE YOUNG BUCKS

Admitting the importance of relationships and communication tools may not be natural for men of our generation. Indeed, men have a well-documented history of not asking for help. However, a look at college campuses today shows that male communication is indeed a genetic possibility and that the stigmas and cultural barriers of older generations need not persist. Two college athletes at St. Lawrence University started an organization called Male Athletes Against Sexual Violence (MAASV) that strived to establish male athletes as a source and responsible group with the moral integrity and courage to speak out against and to protect others from sexual violence. As leaders on the basketball and football team, Rich Williams and Hank Anderson had no problem recruiting young men to their mission. By changing the definition of "alpha-male cool" they attack the problem from within, using facts and open communication to combat an issue that was powered by silence and secrecy. "We can't expect all young men to have confidence," says Williams, "but we want to help them become better men. We can send them forward with a more sophisticated toolbox."

Another group of college guys, more focused on the immediate gratification of open communication, explained how they kept a copy of *Guide to Getting It On*—an indispensable illustrated guide for the sexually curious by Paul Joannides—in their living room. Then they had weekly group and private discussions based on their field trials. This type of tribe provides immediate benefits as well as the basis for a lifelong panel of trusted advisors.

> "Guide to Getting It On is solid in all areas. It's very Pan-sexual."
> —male, age 23

tribes. Any regular outlet is a mental health insurance policy. Be it an athletic event, golf, poker, or bowling night, men would be well-served to create, prioritize, and commit to some venue for communication, in whatever manly guise it must take, and their women would be well-served to encourage them to go—and not give them grief about it. These gatherings need not have a noble purpose. It's about nothing more complicated than not allowing yourself to become isolated from your tribe.

> "It typically involves alcohol and a bonfire . . . or a long hike. I usually end up with more than I wanted to know about my friend and his marriage or problems. Nonetheless, communication is taking place." —male, age 39

TRIBAL MIX

If you don't have logical connections from your past or can't reactivate them, you can still build your panel around who is available. For some of us, panels will require active recruiting of members and, for all of us, panels should be an ever-evolving process. Sometimes the catalyst to deeper understanding lies in perspective from the opposite gender.

Panel members can be loosely related friends who forge a lifelong connection through a shared cause, perfect strangers who meet in a crisis, participants in an intense athletic event, travelers who bond together on a memorable trip, or roommates assigned at random who instantly click. Tribes and panels can coalesce from a variety of places, but you have to invest an open heart and mind to reap the full benefit of the wisdom they provide. Likewise you need to be aware of their limitations. People who already think like you may not challenge you to grow. Save room in your life for scoundrels—the friend or acquaintance who represents the "don't" in every advice column. Pay attention to them in addition to your more upstanding examples as you may just learn some hard emotional lessons on the cheap.

"I think it's very difficult for guys to connect with each other compared to women and their 'girlfriends.' If I have deep stuff to talk about, I find a female colleague or friend. Of all the men I talk with, it's probably easiest with my brother; but in general men aren't good listeners, and I just get frustrated if I need them to listen." —male, age 50

"My two best male friends from college, with whom there has always been a 'why didn't we date' question in the air, are my sounding boards for what is normal in a guy's mind, things like how often do you have sex, who do you think about when you masturbate, are you happy, have you cheated, what drives you crazy in marriage, etc. When I report an argument to my female friends, they usually fully support me and my husband is painted as a complete idiot. But my guys help me see a man's perspective. They also provide a healthy dose of flirting outside of the marriage that serves my middle-agedness well." —female, age 43

Whether your panel is all men or all women or all couples, don't wait until the divorce or the breakup or the affair to seek counsel. It's never too early or too late to build or simply discover your panel. One 55-year-old woman admitted, "I always knew I could talk to my friends about sex but I never knew I could talk to them about not having sex. When I finally opened up about the fact that my husband and I were not having sex and how that made me feel, I started to feel like myself again and had the confidence to get help."

WHAT DO *WE* KNOW?

Cindy: "Growing up the youngest of seven, I was surrounded by sisters and sisters-in-law—my first panel of wise women—who talked about everything from sex drive and childbirth to birth control and body hair. Whatever the issue, they took it on and demystified it for me. By the time I got to actually having sex myself, open communication was my only option. To this day, when I seek out advice from my trusted friends, they share stories of their own, which make me laugh and feel normal and supported. It all started with the original panel."

Edie: "My entire young adult life was spent training, traveling, and competing with a pack of women. Like a big family that knows everything about each other, we were naked in every way. Under the constant pressure of competition, we saw each other at our best and worst. No matter how ugly it got, however, we had nowhere to run. It was great relationship training to learn the value of total and often brutal honesty. Those early uncensored relationships formed a bond that many of us still have today and, now that we're not competing for the same boys, we can talk about sex too, which is handy."

BOTTOM LINE

Women are culturally and socially predisposed to seek out support networks, while men have to make more of an effort to stay connected to their tribes and panels. No gender or age group has a corner on the panel and tribe market—they can save anyone. We think they're the best therapy available.

WHY YOU SHOULD CARE

The fall into silence is a slippery slope in any relationship. If you don't have an outlet to air your questions and vent your frustrations routinely, something is going to give. Panels can offer a wealth of advice and perspective and also take the pressure off your partner to be your sole source of counsel.

WHAT YOU CAN DO

Cultivate and maintain your panel. Reactivate old, meaningful relationships, but also be open to assembling a local panel of friends and mentors you have made in your adult life—particularly ones who you know have seen action on the relationship front you care about yourself. The more you can surround yourself with trusted friends, the more likely you are to get things out in the open and find solutions to problems in your life before they escalate. If you've never had a panel, take the baby step of using the people in this book as a start. They have all shared their triumphs, failures, joys, and frustrations in the spirit of genuinely helping others gain perspective.

It turns me on when he chops wood, is present and engaged with the kids, decreases his alcohol intake, takes care of himself, exercises, watches me undress with the perfect look on his face, and asks me deep questions about myself or about life.
—female, age 42

What turns me on?!? Be in the room with me (we're GUYS for Chrissake—we ALWAYS want to have sex)."
—male, age 41

Real Hot

Sexiness, like beauty, is in the eye of the beholder. What turns people on is relative, but in any healthy relationship it goes beyond straight eye candy. As much as the father of your children may have lusted after the bodacious bathing suit model back in the day, he probably also lusted after flat-chested freckle-faced girls with glasses. Similarly, your wife may have had drive-by dreams of the buffed, deeply tanned construction worker but she didn't really imagine meeting or interacting with that Adonis. Proximity is a huge turn-on, but even more so with reciprocity. There is a universe of things that turn us on and off, including the way we dress, walk, talk, look, smell, behave, move, react . . . as well as where we live, who we know, where we grew up, what we drive, hobbies we like, games we play. The list is endless and personally unique, yet it boils down to a simple constant. If it makes us feel good about ourselves or our partners it's a turn-on.

Our research leads us to this conclusion: sexy is less about how you look and what you wear than the attitudes and actions you put behind it. Nevertheless, as a culture we get hung up on appearances and behaviors that are commonly accepted as alluring, with little regard for whether or not they make us feel attractive or attracted. When attaining the ideal of "hot" takes precedence over appreciating ourselves and our partners for the very qualities that may have brought us together in the first place, we're headed down a road that may completely bypass sexual satisfaction.

HOT LOOKS

Chasing archetypal physical beauty is a black hole for time and energy. Certainly, we all want to look our best, and to be with someone who looks his or her best. But the sexy archetype for women—free of wrinkles, gray hair, body hair, cellulite, panty lines, and all the effects of gravity—is neither attainable nor sustainable for most. Men also can get judged by a checklist of classically sexy attributes, focused more on what they should have than what they're missing: tall, dark, and handsome; six-pack abs; broad, strong chest; full head of hair, full back of no hair. Ideally we would all figure out—before the ring goes on the finger—that the physical attributes we initially perceive as so important are not nearly as important as compatibility in other areas. The man who admits that big boobs and a tight butt may set the hook and even reel him in, also comes to admit those attributes are not solely sufficient to sustain his long-term appetite for intimacy. Similarly, the woman who never thought she could date a guy with a hairy back eventually finds herself unfazed at the somewhat Sasquatch-esque love of her life and repulsed by guys who are vain enough to shave or wax their bodies.

> *I think it's incredibly sexy when a guy is going bald and shears it all off. It says he is confident. The comb-over is unthinkable.*
> —female, age 41

Those who embrace their natural physical attributes optimize them.

HOT DRESS

On the cultural hot-o-meter, dress gets billing directly beneath physical appearance. Men get cut a lot of slack on dress—contractor chic can be dead sexy and a guy in tousled hair and boxers . . . abondanza! But women are bombarded with the message that true beauty requires looking like a lingerie model. Want to know Victoria's "Secret"? Those girls aren't necessarily getting any more action than the girls in Hanes for Her. A man is programmed to believe that buying her lingerie will increase his chances of more sex while women are programmed to believe that men will find them more attractive if they look like underwear models or porn stars. If lingerie in your wife's bureau fuels your—or her—fantasy of possibilities, then it's money well spent. If it reminds you both of inadequacy or unfulfilled desires, it should be removed from the premises with the urgency of a Hazardous Materials team.

One voluptuous beauty, with a strong libido and canyonesque cleavage, assures us that all men like it when you dress up in lingerie, wear heels, and tease them as foreplay. It's likely that most men would like that kind of action if the woman with whom they are engaging in sex had full conviction behind it. But the hitch is in the delivery: show doubt or hesitation and the production is not arousing. For the woman who is comfortable in lingerie and heels, delivering the goods as the vixen in the bedroom gets her man fully charged. Put another woman in that kind of get-up and it can have a completely different effect for a number of reasons. If the woman is not genuinely in that mindset, it can be unsettling for the man to see her uncomfortable and out of her element.

> "When I put lingerie on waiting for my husband to come home, it makes me wet."
> —female, age 48

It's like the comedian who fantasized about a girlfriend stripping for him. When she gave him what he asked for despite her own painfully obvious inexperience in this type of performance, it was the most uncomfortable sexual experience of his life. He felt obligated to enjoy it, but when he unsuccessfully feigned arousal he hurt her feelings. An awkward moment turned into a serious discussion and the expensive lingerie never made it off her body. Be careful what you wish for.

Lingerie is sexy only if the woman is motivated and committed to it making her feel sexy. Some like the feel of it on their skin and get a little lift from having it under their clothes all day. Some women know lingerie turns their husband on so much that it turns them on. Others can't muster a shred of enthusiasm for wearing it. Men are almost uniformly thrilled if their wives are comfortable wearing lingerie, but only if it makes her more randy. A sweaty T-shirt on a body that exudes health and confidence and is game to rumble in the sack is just as sexy. Once again, it's what you put behind it.

> "I received a batch of thongs through an underwear chain letter and worked them into my rotation of otherwise practical underwear. I couldn't tell which end went up when getting dressed for work, predawn. Wearing a thong is highly arousing, especially worn backwards with the thong strap riding your clitoris all day!" —female, age 42

TAKING IT OFF

Reasons for a good trim range from functional to hygienic to cosmetic. Most women need to do some touching up to avoid hair creep beyond the bathing suit, while others require major intervention to prevent their nether regions from fusing into an impenetrable hedgerow. Likewise, certain outfits and certain times of day warrant appropriate underwear. Nonetheless the current hair and pantyline maintenance trends can be baffling. Waxing oneself into prepubescence and wearing thongs exclusively have become such standard behaviors that many people assume they are prerequisites for looking or feeling sexy.

In our quest for enlightenment on this topic, we were interested to learn how some erotic fashions evolved from the efforts of professional strippers hoping to accommodate legal ordinances while still earning big tips. Some states require erotic dancers to wear at least token coverage, hence the thong. It is likewise illegal in some states to show nipples and pubic hair, hence the nipple tassels and full waxing (necessitated by the thong). How these behaviors and attire migrated from the world of strippers and porn stars to the mainstream is somewhat murky, but it is fairly clear that these high-maintenance trends did not debut as solutions for everyday wear.

The Brazilians (the actual people who live in Brazil in case you have forgotten the source) get credit for taking the thong from the realm of the exotic dancer to the beach in the '70s. By the late '80s the thong had crept north to our streets where today—despite the fact that thongs are uncomfortable for many and offer bacteria a rope ladder from your anus to your vagina—it is considered sexy to display exposed anal floss in the back while harboring bald labia up front. Clearly, we have been desensitized to the extreme measures women take to approximate the erotic standards of "sexy," but looking one's age down under is not a commentary on one's desire for sex.

Whether women choose to let the jungle grow, trim it like a putting green, leave a landing strip, or take it all off, what works to support the desires and true comfort of both you and your partner is appropriate. Certainly, any look or feel that makes a woman feel good about herself has positive aspects, but it is just plain sad when women are made to feel self-conscious or embarrassed about showing any natural sign of maturity. Just as getting a Brazilian (the procedure, not a person) and wearing thongs doesn't make one a stripper wannabe, leaving the pubic hair somewhat intact and wearing underwear larger than a banana peel doesn't mean a woman is frumpy, granola-chomping, or prudish. Trust us—two middle-aged women safely outside the realm of conventional hot who have interviewed plenty of women of all ages. The truly, classically hot and "put together" ones, sport varying degrees of pubic hair and underwear coverage. We encourage women to embrace whatever degree makes them feel attractive and comfortable and invite men and women to consider that sexiness can be achieved while still covering your ass.

TAKING IT OFF TAKEN TOO FAR

Once you pare down the underwear, the pubic hair must follow, and once that too is gone the labia are fully exposed, which is—surprise—often not

NOW HAIR THIS: A WORD ON WAXING

By now, many boys and men have been trained that the hairless, marsupial look on women is the norm. Implied in this perception is that there is something inherently unattractive, unclean, and offensive about pubic hair. Although waxing or shaving body and pubic hair is increasingly popular with men—manscaping products account for a mere $8.6 million of the $95.5 million depilatory industry. Women kick in the other $86.9 million. When it comes to pubic hair, most men report that they choose their grooming habits based on how it feels. Especially among athletes, trimming is often purely a matter of comfort. Women, however, and especially young women, feel an expectation to remove all or most of their pubic hair. "You don't want to admit that you don't buy in to waxing as hot," says one female, recent college graduate. "It takes courage to admit you don't wax."

"I agreed to let my husband shave mine off, and afterward I was so pissed. It was ugly down there—one lip was way longer than the other. I almost made him shave his too."
—female, age 37

While waxing can be seen as an innocuous fashion preference, one clear source of the trend is today's inescapable influence of porn. One could argue that porn produces what people want to see, and thus showing less hair is an evolution that reflects the preferences of the average point of view. In this age of heightened pedophilia awareness, it is noteworthy that the porn industry cannot hire or feature underage girls. One way to legally produce the juvenile look for viewers is to replicate it in adult women.

On a practical note, many respectful men point out that weeding through pubic hair can impede the doorbell discovery process, and they extol the benefits of a clean workspace. As one young buck explains, "when there is no hair down there it makes it a little less intimidating, and it's easier to jump in." Likewise, as happens with lingerie, many women—like a pretty sight. This leads to the rise of more cosmetic issues, prompting a growing number of women to undergo labiaplasty, a surgical procedure that cuts through precious erectile tissue to perk up the "lower" lips. Sexologist Betty Dodson cautions all women about the procedure: "Labia plastic surgery is totally unnecessary. The removal of our inner lips is like cutting petals off of flowers. After 30-some years of viewing women's genitals, I can tell you that vulvas with extended inner lips are more abundant than vulvas that look like clam shells. Unfortunately women are too easily brain-

the one who claims she lost her clitoris after her second child but found it after getting a Brazilian bikini wax—do feel sexier with their gear exposed. Points taken, but hair gets a bad rap. Take it off and the clitoris remains hidden under the hood. You still have to lift and separate to get to the goods. Furthermore, there are several theories that suggest pubic hair helps protect a sensitive area from germs and chafe. One gynecologist cautions that the risk of infection that goes along with waxing and shaving is particularly worrisome in such "complicated terrain."

We encourage you to be aware of what motivates your choice and what message you could be sending perhaps unintentionally. Says one 44-year-old mother of two:

"My first full wax turned my husband on and therefore made me feel sexy, but I didn't consider other consequences. For the first time, I found myself uncomfortable enough that I wouldn't undress or even go to the bathroom in front of my children. Inevitably, I will have to answer my kids' questions."

The important thing is that you wear your look with conviction. Be open to new trends but don't be a prisoner to them.

"Hey, if you are intrigued, try it. It is only hair, and it will grow back." —female, age 37

"I did it once and couldn't stand to look at myself in the mirror. I looked like I was 12." —female, age 35

"When you are right up close a full wax looks like a textbook diagram. It's weird. I do like it cleaned up—the last time the full bush was in fashion I was coming out of one—but some hair is perfectly fine." —male, age 23

"Pubes will be back in style, and everyone will be scrambling for merkins." —female, age 77

washed into thinking there is something wrong with the appearance of their sex organs. They fear boyfriends or husbands won't find them sexually appealing."

DEGREES OF HOT

Certainly there is a huge range in what people find attractive and there is enough variety in this world that people have a chance of finding a partner in his/her range of interest. While the prospect of naked sex is all it takes to stimulate some couples, others depend upon an assortment of turn-on accessories from suggestive lingerie or talking dirty to S&M and beyond. What would be considered common daywear on a college campus can be downright incendiary for a couple in their 40s. For some men, seeing their partner in a spaghetti-strap "undershirt" has the same effect as stilettos and a thong for another. An individual's "kinks" are as unique as fingerprints.

> "When my wife wears her tight tank top/leotard thing to bed, I pretty much have to have sex with her. When she talks to her mom just before bed, I pretty much don't want to have sex with her . . . although if she wears the outfit I mentioned, I could overcome it." —male, age 43

In most cases, a little communication about turn-ons and turn-offs can help you find common ground—say, boxers and a fitted T-shirt instead of a full-length flannel nightie.

Before you assemble an arsenal of turn-on gear, be prepared, out of common decency and compassion, to back it up. If the erections in your household are occurring as readily as black flies in May, you might not want to fill your toolbox with erotica, lingerie, and sex toys. For many women cotton underwear is merely a yellow light.

SEXY IS AS SEXY DOES

We've all been there, scratching our heads at "what he sees in her," and "why she's going out with him." We can't emphasize enough that sexy—real sexy—comes from a place much deeper than looks. The radiation of confidence can turn an otherwise ordinary-looking person into a highly desireable sex pot. Ultimately our attraction to someone goes beyond appearance and attire. Behavioral turn-ons are complicated by the way most of us are hardwired at an early age to go after what is bad for us and to desperately pursue whoever will cause us

> "High heels make the legs look great, and make the buttocks infinitely more accessible. That's why Victoria's Secret exists." —male, age 60

> *"I imagine myself as a well-stocked shop that has an open/ closed sign on the front door. When I wear the granny panties the store is closed for business. The fine print actually reads: 'touch me and I'll break your arm and beat you with the bloody stump.' If, when my husband peeks under the covers, I have the sexy, lacy little thong undies on, the store is most definitely open for business. Occasionally, the store is closed but the door is unlocked, indicating the proprietress could be persuaded to extend her hours. For these occasions, the half-lacy, half-Hanes undies are the sign."* —female, age 43

the most heartache, the most work, and the least return for our effort. Any of us have fallen for the High Maintenance Factor at one time or another, for the hot, emotionally distant partner who blows us off at every turn, then throws us a booty call when they're between relationships.

Men reflect on their younger years as a time when they were turned on by one type of girl, but actually wanted long-term relationships with a different type. Women reflect on how much those guys pissed them off. Dating is unendingly frustrating for the girl who is "the kind guys want to marry, not date," and for the nice guy who is "just friends" to all the girls. Eventually, high maintenance and unavailability lose their appeal while adoration and devotion become immensely attractive. We come to value most, the people who make us feel good without the torture.

WHAT DO *WE* KNOW?

Edie: "I knew this guy for months in the city and we occasionally met up for drinks, but never even kissed each other good night and were not the least bit attracted to each other 'that way.' One night after dinner, he hopped in the taxi, again with no kiss and for some reason the thought just popped into my head: 'That's someone I'm never going to sleep with.' Ten years and two kids later, I can safely say I was wrong. It all turned around when we went skiing together by chance. Once we saw each other in our respective comfort zones doing something we both loved to do we were incredibly attracted to each other."

Cindy: "For decades people have been giving me unsolicited advice on how to turn men on and how to be more feminine. I stopped listening at age 22, and my sex life has thrived ever since. It seems to me that the most important thing about underwear is that they are off while we are having healthy, open sex."

KNOW WHEN TO TURN IT OFF

One man insists that his wife tell him kinky stories about herself, which she willingly makes up. This works fine for them but seems to be a bit of an outlier. When people say talking dirty is a turn-on, for the most part they are referring to urgent requests and direction in the heat of the moment that indicate desire, as in, "I want you in me now!" and not necessarily hugely graphic adult bedtime scripts.

Some couples tell each other their fantasies or watch sexy movies together. These types of turn-ons have to be mutual—at least understood and accommodated—or they can backfire. Many things arouse us in theory but not in reality. As one young man who tried to replicate pornographic acts with his girlfriend concluded, "Some things are just better off left for masturbation fuel." Desire to please your partner is a turn-on but being overly desirous and behaving like a starved animal can work against you.

"I dated one guy and in the heat of the moment he said, 'I want to lick your clit until you die.' I couldn't believe it at first. Then I burst out laughing. The relationship pretty much ended at that point."
—female, age 42

COMFORT IS KEY

The classic tales of long-time friends suddenly falling in love with each other, or of a women progressively turning her affections to her boyfriend's roommate, attest that comfort—with ourselves and with each other—can be a powerful and sustaining turn-on. Close on its heels are willingness and proximity.

"I really appreciate when my wife is willing to have sex just because she knows that it has been a while, But it doesn't turn me on as it does when I know that she really wants to have sex."
—male, age 44

Most men are turned on by whatever it is that makes a woman more interested in sex, and most of all by being desired. Conversely, offering mercy sex is SO not a turn-on. Men tell us that the chief attraction of porn and strippers is the idea that the women are enjoying the act. The responsiveness is the turn-on. Women take note—turning someone on can be as straightforward as allowing yourself to be turned on, and then of course showing it.

Guys, remember, the pros are getting paid for that. You may need to reconsider if you want the mother of your children to develop an act.

Feeling good about yourself can make you more attractive. Any little step you make toward improving your health can have immediate positive effects on your mindset and the energy you put out there. Physical activity then, has huge potential. When we exercise, we feel good about ourselves, we generally look better, and we exude a degree of health and confidence. Some research suggests that people are attracted to each other's smells, which are undoubtedly accentuated during physical activity. One woman was so smitten by watching her then-boyfriend play football at Thanksgiving that she had sex with him that night in his parent's home. "I was so turned on by watching him in the football game, I went for it. After 10 years of marriage I still barely do that in their home."

> *"I just want a little feedback. It could be words or noises, moans, grunts, contact, touching, whatever will do it."*
> —male, age 27

BOTTOM LINE

The ultimate goal is to have communication, humor, and enjoyment in your sex life. Embrace what you've got. If it makes you and your partner feel good, do it, wear it, and say it.

WHY YOU SHOULD CARE

Despite what our culture and the media feed us constantly, being truly hot is immediately attainable for us all.

WHAT YOU CAN DO

Don't get hung up on looks. In the long run, looks neither handicap you nor grant you a "Get out of Jail Free" card. Do focus on confidence and communication. No matter who you are, those are your best assets.

Women: You don't have to look, dress, or act like a stripper to be sexy. Just because a guy squirrels away Victoria's Secret catalogs for his own private entertainment doesn't mean he is any less attracted to his wife, or needs her to look and behave like one of those models. Of course, if some of that spice is grounded in mutual respect for each other, Game On! The biggest turn-on you can offer a man is to show you desire him.

Men: Occasionally you may need a little reminder that the hunger, exhaustion, and silicone required to maintain the conventional ideal of beauty can be a waste of time and energy and, sometimes self-esteem. Putting each other at ease will bring out the heat in both of you.

THE LIFECYCLE OF TURN-ONS

Turn-ons change as our lives change, which is good news and bad. High school guys can have, conservatively, six or seven boners a day in response to anything vaguely attractive, like the way the curve of the teacher's hip looks when she writes on the board, or for no reason at all—the so-called NORB (No Reason Boner). From that state of carbonation, we go to the opposite end of the spectrum, to the post-partum female with an infant on her hip and toddler underfoot, for whom sleep is the single biggest turn-on. The bad news is that the trenches of family life are anything but erotic. The good news is that even in the darkest moments of your sex life, getting turned on is more simple and attainable than what the media suggests.

TURN-ONS FOR MEN

Generally men need little coaxing to get in the mood for sex, as is evidenced by their answers to what things women can do to turn them on. They rarely get beyond a few words like showing up, breathing, getting naked, being friendly, and making an effort to look nice. More than that, feeling appreciated and desired are sure-fire turn-ons.

"The biggest turn-on is having your wife pull off your underwear, part your lips with her tongue, and tell you to pull off her nightgown while she helps wiggle out of her panties." —male, age 43

"Before I was having great sex I fantasized about women who look sexed up. Now I fantasize about women who are ready and primed regardless of what they look and dress like. Big tits when you are younger are HOT. Now I look at a woman and wonder if she enjoys sex and that is hot."
—male, age 23

TURN-ONS FOR WOMEN

Beyond the standard list of private time without kids, dinner out, back rubs, helping with chores, being spontaneously affectionate, going away for the weekend, and the occasional flowers, are other efforts that get women in the mood.

"When he takes care of his body—doesn't drink too much or eat crappy food—he is more attractive to me."
—female, age 42

"Having dinner made when I get home is a HUGE turn on. Thoughtfulness, period, that does it for me."
—female, age 42

"I like sleep a lot and apparently I will do anything for it, including having sex when I am dead tired at night so I can sleep those 10 extra minutes in the morning."
—female, age 37

"I am most excited about sex when there are no kids, there is no phone, and we are on vacation." —female, age 34

"If there was an option for sex after lunch with no kids, and I could have a nap to follow, that would be an ideal sex situation."
—female, age 35

TURN-OFFS FOR MEN

Even though men are usually eager for sex, a little reciprocation and appreciation will go a long way, and a lack of it can be, well, withering.

"I do not appreciate feeling like a walking ATM that does heavy lifting around the house. What's the fun in that?" —male, age 48

"The biggest turn-off is when my wife makes the kids more important than the marriage." —male, age 43

"Leaving me to clean up the post-dinner mess and make lunches while she's chatting on the phone or checking email—that shoots down the intimate side of things."
—male, age 41

TURN-OFFS FOR WOMEN

It should come as no big surprise that being rude or bossy, drinking too much, or pressuring her or whining for sex are not turn-ons.

"Lack of communication is a turn-off. He works long hours and often gets home when I am asleep or too exhausted to hash out any issues at hand. So tough." —female, age 43

"It kind of kills the mood when he blows his nose, smells bad, has Caesar salad or garlic for dinner, farts as he gets in to bed, or stinks up the bathroom right before coming to bed." —female, age 39

"At the end of the day I am so over the caregiving role. I can't handle a needy man at that point." —female, age 37

"Good sex is all about vulnerability. If you are constantly acting, you are not in the moment. It's not true intimacy unless you can let your guard down."
—female, age 37

"There is no such thing as 'good in bed.' Communication skills are good in bed. Women blame men all the time, but it is often their fault for not speaking up and telling guys what they like."
—male, age 23

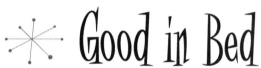

Good in Bed

Thanks to movies and other media, we get the message that being good in bed requires some sort of advanced degree, special talent, superior physical attributes, or triple-X rating. The Hollywood version of good lovin', while it may lead to arousal, is rarely educational on how to actually please a partner and almost never portrays the courage it takes to ask for guidance. It also promotes the erroneous expectation that great lovers innately know how to please.

WHAT DO WE KNOW?

Cindy: "When I was younger, I thought there were people who were just plain good in bed because they were so skilled. In my mind, attractive people with their unlimited access to other attractive people got more practice and therefore had more useful sex information. When you are hot, you must be a pro who gets experience with and information from other pros. It turns out that there is not a secret society of sex gods and goddesses. In fact most hot people don't get much information or guidance because anyone climbing in the sack with those people assumes what I assumed: they know it all. The hot people are actually left in the dark more than the regular people."

Edie: "When I was in my 20s and had just started having sex, I worried out loud to a friend over whether or not I was good in bed. She looked at me like I was an idiot and exclaimed, 'You have a hole don't you!?!' At that stage of life, considering the immediate needs of the guys in my life, she was probably right."

WHO IS GOOD IN BED?

Placing "good in bed" on a pedestal not only can make us insecure in our own abilities to please each other, but can also emphasize the performance aspect of sex. Feelings of inadequacy or anxiety over our lovemaking skills only widens the space between partners. The helpful message to understand is that we can all be good in bed if we are having sex with someone with whom we are connected through mutual attraction and trust. With those two elements, each partner should have the courage, comfort, and motivation to ask questions, have sex unselfconsciously, and seek the information that leads to truly good sex.

BEDDING BASICS

It's true that our bodies are wired for doing what comes naturally. Womens' bodies respond and encourage through early-to-mid-level arousal, but often that automatic feedback process stops when we are only halfway to the goal line. Getting most women to orgasm requires some navigating, trial and error, and guidance. It's safe to say that pleasing a woman can be a challenge—we will address some of the reasons later in the book where we focus on orgasms.

Meanwhile, giving a healthy man an orgasm is sort of like boiling water. Adding salt can make it quicker, it takes longer at altitude, and sometimes it's hard to get the fire lit, but keep at it long enough and eventually, it's going to happen. Given the relative ease with which most men reach orgasm (moisture + warmth + friction), one might assume that it's not too challenging for women to be good in bed. Even the horniest men assure us, however, that a lifetime of making love to a minimally responsive warm body is unsatisfactory. What takes sex from being just okay to being good or even great starts with a strong partner connection that fosters openness and responsiveness.

MAKING YOUR BED

The art of being good in bed starts well outside of the bedroom. It begins by creating the feeling of comfort that comes when sex is the expression of the emotional connection rather than the source. One working mother of three finds herself unable to touch base with her husband in a meaningful way as they scramble through the work week. "If we don't really talk and listen to each other during the week and lay in bed not speaking for five nights straight, then having sex on the sixth day isn't going to keep us connected. It makes me so mad when he thinks that sex is the thing that is going to make us connect. For me, the connection comes before the sex, not during." If you communicate in other areas of your relationship it is not much of a leap to do it in your intimate life. If you do not communicate well elsewhere, the bedroom can be a loaded place to start, especially considering that men tend to use physical intimacy as a vehicle to emotional connection while most women crave emotional connection to be motivated for physical intimacy. We'll talk more about this logjam in Section 3, but suffice it to say that both sides need to give a little on this point.

As you review your sexual highlight reel, you may be smirking and skeptical about one thing. If good sex is all about connection, what explains the unbridled pleasure of the one-night stand? Certainly we hear time and again, that the absolute best sex people ever had was during a wild, uninhibited one-night stand, where both partners had superhuman stamina. Our thinking is that one-night-stand sex may be so outrageously good because of the connection of intent, in this case the "intent" being not to connect. Neither person is burdened by the other's complicated past nor intimidated by the prospect of an uncertain future. But it is a short-lived pleasure, typically accompanied the next day by some form of "walk of shame," and the clearheaded realization that, for relationships to last more than one night, you can't really de-couple from sex. Even if that one-night stand turns into a lasting relationship, the disconnectedness that fueled that athletic, hedonistic sex is replaced by the slow simmer of reality sex, which, as we mature, is all most of us can handle emotionally. Indeed, great or mind-blowing sex with a long-term partner can be so physically and emotionally exhausting that, for some, it requires inner reserves of energy. What is exhilarating and tantalizingly memorable in the one-night stand, is unsustainable in the scheme of a long-term relationship where, for many, good sex is just, well, having sex.

IT'S NOT ALL ABOUT YOU

One European woman we interviewed was quick to point out that men from cultures that pride themselves on being great lovers are, in fact, often the worst. This is less about nationality than ego. Pleasing the woman becomes an egocentric act when the man is so invested in his "success" that he is unreceptive to the signals his partner is sending him about what she wants or needs. "They (nationality withheld) aren't the sex gods they are made out to be . . . it's true that they don't have too many inhibitions, but they think way too much about themselves and their sexual skills and what women are supposedly looking for." Another woman recalls dating an attractive self-assured man who didn't bother communicating verbally because he prided himself on his ability to make love to women with his eyes. "If I could have blindfolded him the sex would have been much better. As it was, he creeped me out." Casanovas take note—deep, meaningful eye contact works great in the movies but can be unsettling in real life, even among close couples.

Good in bed is not a static state of being, but a fluid skill of adaptation. One man recalls his initial success as a young buck giving his girlfriend an orgasm. "I struck gold with my hand the first time out." Then he had a girlfriend who was anatomically lined up to easily have orgasms during intercourse. "I figured I was just really good in bed." And he was, for her. Then he moved on to new partners, and it wasn't clear if it was working for them, but they didn't speak up or offer any feedback. "I just went with the harder and faster technique to be sure. And now looking back I am sure they weren't having orgasms." In fact, such bursts of vitality, however well-intentioned, may be counterproductive if not accompanied by some sign of encouragement. At a certain level of arousal, the vaginal cavity expands and a cul de sac opens up above the cervix. That's when a woman may give you the "all clear" to hammer away.

> "If he asked me what to do I'd tell him everything."
> —female, age 27

GOOD SEX IS . . . BAD SEX IS . . .

Everybody has his or her own idea about what constitutes good sex. Short and sweet, uninterrupted, communicative, fun and playful, relaxed and unhurried, cozy, gentle, and athletic are some of the many ways people describe good sex.

Bad sex owes itself to a variety of factors, from vaginal dryness or fatigue to feeling rushed, unappreciated, annoyed, or fat. One consistent answer from men and women is that bad sex is selfish.

> "I wish she'd tell me what she liked but I don't dare ask because I think I'm supposed to know." —male, age 27

Patience is a virtue, especially in bed. Being good in bed doesn't end with your own resolution. One woman notes with displeasure, "Once he has been drained, he is indifferent. He is no longer hyperfocused on getting what he needs, so to some extent, he becomes

MYTHS AND REALITY

MYTH: BIGGER IS BETTER, MALE VERSION.

REALITY: They vary wildly in length, angle, shape, head size, etc. The erect version of a penis is often very different than the limp state. Heterosexual guys who only see other erect penises in porn (where oversized penises are as much the norm as oversized breasts) often feel inadequate about penis size even though that perception is warped. There are growers (that start small and get significantly bigger) and showers (that start large and only get a little bigger). Bottom line is they all work. Furthermore, women are more concerned with the way a man uses his penis than its size. Some well-endowed men accessorize their units with a sense of entitlement; they expect women to dance around the maypole while they lie back and add little or no effort to the lovemaking process. Some of the most orgasmic sex reported to us by women came from the guys sporting small penises. As the second-place rental car agency says, "We Try Harder," and we all know it's the thought that counts.

MYTH: BIGGER IS BETTER, FEMALE VERSION.

REALITY: Hooters exists for a reason. Large breasts are magnets for male attention and fantasy. But up close and personal, its not the size of the breast but the responsiveness of the nipple that is erotic. People overstate the role of breast size in the pleasure department and underestimate the power of the nipple.

MYTH: MODEL GIRLS HAVE MODEL SEX.

REALITY: Model girls have the same sex as the rest of us, if they're lucky. Some of the hottest-looking girls are so inwardly focused on staying hot that they can't possibly give or receive pleasure freely.

MYTH: ONE-NIGHT STANDS ARE THE GREATEST COUP SINCE FREE NACHOS AT HAPPY HOUR.

REALITY: Nothing is free and no-strings-attached sex doesn't exist. Somebody gets burned and neither party feels "good" the next day. As a rule of thumb, and this applies to everything you deliberate about during daylight—from sex with a new partner, to phone calls, food, or online purchases: If it sounds like a good idea at 11 p.m., it's not. Lack of communication and connection leads you straight into the walk of shame, the coyote arm, and weeks of torturously unreturned messages to you or from you.

MYTH: ALL MEN THINK BLOW JOBS ARE BETTER THAN SEX.

REALITY: Believe it or not, some actually do not like them and many men say they are over-rated. "Blow jobs are like caviar or fois gras—they can be outrageously good but you can't live on them." As with every other love act, oral sex is best when it's genuine. It's nice to feel like a porn star, but not at the expense of feeling like a charity case.

MYTH: ALL WOMEN LIKE TO RECEIVE ORAL SEX.

REALITY: While oral sex is the expressway to orgasms for some, it is awkward to the point of being unpleasant for others. "When I think of how it must smell down there, even when I'm clean, it makes me cringe." Some women simply don't like the turn-taking aspect of oral sex. "I don't want someone to go down on me so I can come first. I like fucking!"

MYTH: THE MOST EXPERIENCED LOVERS ARE THE BEST LOVERS.

REALITY: True, practice makes perfect, but all the practice in the world won't get you better without a willingness to respond to feedback. Approach sex like an explorer rather than a hunter and you'll learn from your adventures rather than just putting a notch in the bedpost.

MYTH: ONCE A STALLION ALWAYS A STALLION.

REALITY: Times change, so do partners. What works on one won't necessarily work on another. What works one day may not work the next day. As they say on Wall Street: "Past performance is no guarantee of future results."

MYTH: FEMALE ORGASMS NEED TO HAPPEN EVERY TIME.

REALITY: Be careful not to put the cart before the horse. Connection and communication are the elements that open the door to let it happen. The stress on women to have an orgasm and on men to give them can slow or stall the journey for you both. For women, having an orgasm may not always be necessary to enjoy a sexual experience.

MYTH: SIMULTANEOUS ORGASMS ARE THE HOLY GRAIL.

REALITY: Its nice when the stars align, but added pressure can actually lower your odds of colliding. It's a whole lot of work for a marginal benefit that doesn't last much beyond the moment. It's the cherry on top, not the sundae.

MYTH: OYSTERS ARE APHRODISIACS.

REALITY: Okay, here's one that's true! Oysters are high in zinc, which is often low in men who have sexual dysfunction. Bone up on your zinc with pumpkin seeds and pine nuts and oats, which along with zinc provide protein and minerals needed to produce healthy seminal fluids. No wonder the Quaker guy looks so smug.

GOOD BEDIQUETTE

You don't need to be psychic to anticipate your partner's needs. Common sense and little touches of kindness that put your partner at ease are always appropriate and appreciated.

- If you sense your partner is feeling nervous or overly exposed, turn out the light. Says one very yoga-licious 45-year-old woman: "After 40 it's lights out."
- If hearing noise or making noise is a distraction to your partner, shut the door and keep the primal noisemaking as low as you can.
- Focus on the objective. Turn off the TV, your cell phone—your Blackberry, for God's sake. In fact, get rid of all electronics or at least those that are not actively serving your purpose of intimacy.
- Finish what you start. Blue balling isn't just for guys. True, getting there is half the fun, but only if you actually get there.
- Feign interest after the act, or at least don't fall asleep when still engaged.
- Have a moment. Don't jump up immediately when the deed is done to shower, mop up, find your book, etc. Make yourself count to 20 if you have to. If the wet spot is going to torture your laundry reflex put a towel beside the bed. Put it underneath you if it's that big a deal.
- Take the pressure off. It may be better to look away, close your eyes, or turn out the light. Also, asking for progress reports can feel too intense.

aloof." In general, the speed differential between men and women requires men to have more patience in the process of bringing women to climax. Women, in turn, need to understand what men are up against and be patient with their attempts to please. Both partners need to approach sex with a genuine desire to learn what pleases each other and the acknowledgment that neither of you is psychic.

Finally, what's good for you may be what makes you good in bed. Sex studies show that looking out for number one—that is, taking responsibility for your own pleasure rather than depending on your partner for sense of self, reassurance, and approval—is arousing to your partner. If you deal with your own emotions first, instead of laying that burden on your partner, you're better able to please and be pleased.

BOTTOM LINE

It is the connection and the feeling of being at ease that makes someone good in bed. Mechanics are important but only effective if they work in concert with the good dynamics you create.

WHY YOU SHOULD CARE

Being good in bed isn't a badge of honor, but it is a hefty incentive to incorporate good communication skills into your relationship.

WHAT YOU CAN DO

Focus on connection rather than performance. Once you have the connection with your partner, encourage discussion and communication about what turns you on. By being open about what you're feeling you'll find that some "skills" are no-brainers. (Case in point: lube, lube lube! Be it a scoop of KY or a dab of Astroglide, it'll set you free.) Bodies change, moods change—there is no one technique that works every time so approach sex as an organic exploration rather than a set of mechanical tasks. Performance hitches a ride on connection.

♀ / ♂

"Doggie style is completely out of the question for me— too much junk in the trunk."
—female, age 41

"This body image stuff drives men nuts. We don't understand it because we don't dwell much on our own body images. Look, once we have chosen you of course we want you to try to stay fit and look good. But when it comes to sex we care a whole lot less about your body than you think, as long as you are willing to rub it up against us!" —male, age 39

Iceberg Ahead: The Vicious Cycle of Body Image

Negative female body image—not the way a woman looks but the way she "feels" she looks—is probably the most treacherous territory for couples when it comes to communicating their respective intimacy needs. This issue often comes to the fore after children. Women and men need to recognize body image for what it is in the female psyche. It is the iceberg that can bring down even the Titanic of sexual desire. Consider the dynamic that fuels the following no-win scenarios:

Scenario 1: Woman shuns intimacy because she feels unattractive. Man offers suggestions—diet or a gym membership or a beauty treatment—that in his mind, will logically address her problems. Those suggestions validate the woman's body insecurities, making her feel even less desirable to, and desirous of, her man.

Scenario 2: Man compliments woman on positive aspects of her appearance and she stores those compliments in her vault. When her weight fluctuates, her hair grays, her breasts sag, or she feels various signs of wear, she

"Are you waiting to be skinnier, thinner, more toned, more tanned, better dressed, sexier, more lovable, nicer, smarter, funnier, or wealthier before you really begin your life? Millions of us are. And it's a complete waste of time. Body obsession and the quest for perfection are destroying our lives, and we are willing partners in this destruction."

—Jessica Wiener, in *Do I look fat in this?* (Simon and Schuster)

retrieves those compliments to feel comparatively undesirable, and thereby turns the man's own compliments against him.

One perceptive 44-year-old man describes the familiar downward spiral: "Negative body image drives down the woman's desire or appetite for sex. Because guys tend to overlook or forget that their spouses may feel this way, they start thinking that it is a personal attack on them when they initiate sex and get turned down because of her lack of desire. In reality it is just her negative feelings overruling desire. Then she adds guilt to her unhappiness and he feels rejected, which over time may drive down his desire to keep trying."

Love is cruel! How do we stop the madness? Women know it is irrational, destructive, and immature, but it's there and the best we can do is warn you from the crow's nest. Men who learn to navigate around the iceberg's immovable power will pass unscathed, and get a lot more of what they want.

ICEBERG AWARENESS

A women doesn't see herself through the eyes of her partner. Too often she appraises herself in the mirror, one piece at a time. Whatever she sees depends on more factors than anyone outside her own brain could ever contemplate, many of them buried in childhood and adolescence, then reinforced through life experiences, social hierarchies, and our culture. In every piece, she sees what she wants to be, what she could be, what she used to be, and very rarely, happily accepts what she is. To her man, her body may be a wonderland, but to her it is at best a work in progress. When mood and hormones conspire to make her especially sensitive to the iceberg's heft—the butt she thinks is too big, the breasts she thinks are too small, the belly that reminds her of a baggy skinned mastiff—many areas cease to function as erogenous zones. They are her own battle zones, so approach them with care. Hold back your comments and judgments because even positive comments can backfire.

Men, you may not be responsible for creating this natural hazard, and you certainly can't be responsible for getting rid of it, but you don't have to contribute to its growth. As a culture, we are bombarded with media images from fashion models, celebrities, and ads that define and celebrate a narrow image of female physical perfection. Women learn to index their inherent attractiveness and desirability to unnatural standards of weight, body type, breast size, hair color, skin tone and tautness, etc. The reasons we do this—whether cultural, parental, or societal—are the stuff around which self-help empires are built and beyond the scope of this book. What you need to know, fellas, is that your seemingly logical suggestion of a diet or gym membership, however innocent, becomes an endorsement of those standards in your woman's mind. Suggest cosmetic surgery or Botox and you are really getting to be part of the larger societal problem.

Women, surely there are times we wish a size 6 figure, perky C-cups, peaches-and-cream skin, or a figure skater's butt were part of our natural raw materials. But we don't get to write our own DNA and lamenting it will not make us attractive.

What will make us attractive is how we think more realistically and positively about ourselves. We have found that husbands out there generally aren't concerned with a 10-to-15-pound weight swing. Sure, they notice it—we would accuse them of being oblivious if they didn't—but it's

ICEBERG COMMENTARY FROM A SALTY CAPTAIN

"The body image thing drives me freaking nuts. In brief: women are body-obsessed for themselves (and also for other women) NOT for their partners, especially AFTER marriage. I don't know one husband amongst my good friends and casual beer buddies who cares a fig about his wife's weight. I would venture a vast, vast, majority of men would rather have their mates carry an extra 10–15 pounds and not be crabby than be svelte and always be fighting a diet depression. Men have a much greater tolerance for their long-term partners' weight than given credit for.

"Admittedly, men are fools for looks when dating, opting for the dumb hottie over the chubby smartie every time. But once a guy is locked into a relationship, it's all about having a happy wife/happy life. You see, when a wife has a bad day, the whole house has a bad day. And when a wife is obsessed with looking like skinny Cameron Diaz, there are a lot of bad days. Husbands shell out a lot of money to cover wives' gym memberships, home workout equipment, expensive fad diets, and so on, NOT so their wives can lose weight, but because husbands know if their wives get no deal killer. Take it from this wise father of three: "My wife has kids. Her body changes. She liked her old body. I liked the old one too. I also like the new one, and the pregnant one. I just want to have sex with my wife, whatever her shape. A little extra weight—still hot. A few more wrinkles—no problem. Bags under her eyes—don't worry, I'll be quick so she can get back to sleep."

What's a guy to do? Encouraging words about her beautiful body can be a waste of time. In fact, they do more harm than good. You could hold your tongue and wait for your wife to develop a positive body image, but that might never happen. If you encourage your wife to do something about it—jog, walk, anything—you're opening up a can of worms. The problem is when you say "you should go jogging," your wife hears "you need to lose weight." The truth is, you want her to jog so she feels better about herself and gets back to being horny. Generally, men are much better at confining their body image to the physical realm, while women let emotions dictate how they look. When women are feeling low or weak, they don't take good care of themselves. Says one woman, "This is when we need support from men, and the one way we can help guys help us is to talk about it with them. They can't read our minds and so we have to guide them from the beginning. We need to be able to say, 'look, I'm not feeling 100 percent, I could use use a little extra positives at this time.'"

in shape, they will be easier to live with. So the weight loss actually is a secondary goal, not the primary goal.

"The subtext in all of this body-image nonsense is that women need to feel good about their bodies and their appearances to feel sexy. The better women feel about how they look, the more likely they are to put out. Consequently, husbands indirectly become enablers for their wives body-obsession NOT because they insist their wives look like Cameron Diaz (though that would be fine), but because they want happy wives who put out. Husbands intuitively know that the physical stuff is a losing proposition due to the aging process, so it's a battle that their wives can't possibly win.

"The Grand Unified Theory of Marriage that wives don't get is that pretty much all sex is good sex for husbands. Their wife's physical appearance (within reason) is greatly immaterial. A lot of husbands get really peeved with their wives' obsession with body image because it drives their wives loony. Husbands want happy, not loony, wives because happy is way better than loony—and happy means more sex. And that, my friend, makes the world go round." —slightly bitter male, age 48

IMAGE IS EVERYTHING

The real turn-off is not the post-kids body, or simply post-prime body, but the way that change manifests itself in a woman's own self-image. Women say "I feel that extra layer of insulation on me and it makes me want to cover up," or "I hate it when he squeezes my fat," or "I wish he'd quit staring at my ass," or "How can he think I am sexy when I feel so gross?"

Meanwhile men tell us that the most attractive women are the ones who are comfortable with themselves. One woman, married 10 years, tells how much her sex life has improved since she lost 20 pounds, yet admits that it has nothing to do with her husband's view of her or her weight. "He truly didn't care about the weight, but now that I feel sexier I dress sexier and act sexier. It's all connected." Conversely, when a woman does not feel good about her body, she tends to do things that make her feel and act less sexy. One woman who admittedly does not have a "problem" with her weight, nonetheless explains: "When I am thin for me, I feel sexy, wear tight jeans and a thong. If I am a few pounds up, I untuck my shirt and put on my Hanes Her Ways."

A great body is not a panacea for our hang-ups. One extremely fit, attractive, and experienced single man, when presented with the prospect of a strikingly attractive woman, immediately dismissed the prospect of dating her based on a photograph. He took one look at her ripped abs and sculpted shoulders and said, "She's a Body Nazi. Been there before, and I don't want to get involved with that." Whether or not you want to project a distress signal, getting overly obsessed with your body sends up a red flag.

WHAT IS IT WORTH TO YOU?

Men who make appearance of prime importance need to know what they're asking for. Some women are naturally blessed with slender bodies and others enjoy and take pride in the ongoing activities that support a fit boy. However, the relentless pursuit of "a look" too often creates a neurotic, obsessive woman whose appearance is an all-consuming priority. She is so hungry for whatever it is that is not feeding her soul, and her criticism is so inwardly focused that sharing her body joyfully is a near impossibility. If that's what you want, understand the compromises that go along with making physical appearance the number-one priority of your relationships.

Women need to learn to give men the benefit of the doubt. Accept the possibility that he is attracted to the whole package of you. There are other aspects of the relationship on which he would prefer you spend your energy and attention. Furthermore, he is most likely less critical of you than you are of yourself.

When he caresses you he is likely not feeling your fat or casting judgment on your curves or lack thereof. Not all men lust after the skinny model types. As one woman says, "Most real men I know think the bony thing is nasty." Some men actually prefer it when a woman is on the upper edge of her weight range. "I love her 'mama' body," says one husband.

Of course, if the perfect body really is a condition of his love, don't expect him to support you in anything other than appearances. Better to learn that sooner than later. Women whose partners routinely make them feel bad about their bodies and appearance need to lose a lot of weight—we're talking permanently—but that involves a lawyer, a hit-man, or advice beyond our scope.

A LITTLE GOES A LONG WAY

It doesn't take much physical activity or mental space to start feeling better, and often you can squeeze a lot into very small spaces of time. Sometimes women are uncomfortable asking for the time they need to do something just for them. They feel so out of shape or overweight or run down that even envisioning how they'll get back to a good space is a task. But almost as soon as you make a change, the benefits kick in. One woman who had two babies in quick succession remembers how little it disrupted her husband's schedule to get the time she needed for herself. "I got up to work out before the kids got up. It cost him 20 minutes of taking charge of the kids in the morning and made me feel 100 percent better." Most men can agree in theory to their wives making time for themselves, but the men that proactively make time are the most helpful.

THE BIG PICTURE

Women and men both need to understand that soul-satisfying sex for the long haul comes from appreciating and providing a more diverse menu of attributes than the killer body. Think of the food pyramid, and of how long you could survive on marshmallows and martinis alone.

In the larger scheme, remember that a father's attitude is key in the early female years. If fathers are respectful of their daughters and reinforce positive body

"I realize that my partner does not look like the SI swimsuit issue model, but that does not diminish my desire in the least bit. We had great sex when she was pregnant, and man was her body different then." —male, age 43

image, the chances are better that as women they will choose men who are respectful. Sons who grow up with a father who appreciates women for what's on the inside are more likely to do the same. Mothers have an enormous impact on their daughters and their lifelong body image issues. When daughters see their mothers constantly dieting and lamenting their own bodies, they get the message to do the same.

WHAT DO *WE* KNOW?

Cindy: "Even though I am no petite flower—my muscles and layer of frosting are in full force—I have never had body-image issues. It traces pretty clearly back to my dad. When my siblings and I called my mom fat, he'd say, 'Your mother is healthy. You've got to have meat on your bones!' Of the women who obsessed about their weight he warned: 'Do *not* be like them, wasting their time and energy sitting around talking about calories and diets.' Once when a guy commented on my sports-scarred knees my dad spoke right up. 'That's because she lives her life!' If there's one thing he taught me it is to live in my body and be grateful for everything it is capable of doing."

Edie: "I am without a doubt the iceberg queen. I know it's irrational, not to mention irritating, but I've spent a lifetime honing this insecurity and it's not going anywhere. Feeling fat can blow my day, or be an excuse to dig myself a really deep pit. Weight—wanting to lose it or not wanting to gain it—affects me in some way every day. The best I can do is to be aware of it and up front about it. I came into my relationship with this chronic condition fully disclosed and my husband deals with it masterfully. Every so often when he has to talk me off the edge of the iceberg he skips trying to get me to appreciate my body and instead says something to the effect of: 'You always look hot to me, but you look best when you feel good about yourself.' The message not only melts me a bit, but also puts it in my court to take whatever actions will help me stop obsessing."

BOTTOM LINE

There is an old joke that asks how to please a woman and how to please a man. As you might guess, the women's conditions are long and complicated, some of them having nothing to do with sex or romance. The men's conditions are simply: Show up naked.

Really, it's that complicated. A smile helps.

WHY YOU SHOULD CARE

Men: The fastest way to keep her from wanting to have sex is by making her feel self-conscious about her body.

Women: Your obsessions get tiresome to men, no matter how understanding they are. Eventually, if you dwell on your inadequacies too much you may be creating a new relationship negative. It won't show up in the mirror but in the long run it can be far more debilitating than a crooked smile, an extra inch, or a padded rear end. However caveman-like it sounds, men are attracted to women who give themselves freely. You can't give if you're shrinking away from yourself. Likewise your body isn't inviting if you are overly invested in its fortress-like strength.

WHAT YOU CAN DO

Men: Expect the iceberg and don't try to ram through it. Navigate around it. Show acceptance and compassion on her bad days. Turn out the light, let her get to the bed without checking her out, and warm her up by touching something in more neutral territory than the usual hot spots. Think outside of the box, so to speak. The most sensitive sexual areas are the breasts, nipples, genitals, and lips as well as the ear lobes, fingers, and toes. The soft skin inside the elbows and knees, the small of the back, and the nape of the neck are also in the zones. Foot rub anyone?

Women: Recognize that your iceberg is your own creation. Be open and talk about how you feel, not in an endlessly whining way, but as a way to let him know how you struggle with it. Once in the open your troubles will feel easier, and may even become a source of bonding amusement to you both. Openness can create an avenue for expression and gratitude for the aspects of your body you do appreciate. This alone can help shift your mindset. If you are in a zone beyond the reach of gratitude, try "out of sight, out of mind" for a while. Move the scales and full-length mirrors from your daily beat or try on a little disguise, like this woman did: "The other night I decided to put on this lace teddy that snaps at the crotch. My husband unsnaps the crotch and the lovely lace teddy covers my stomach so I do not have to be turned off by looking at my belly—I just see the sexy lace."

If you want to lose weight or get in shape, by all means go for it with gusto and with support. If you can't commit to that regimen, get over it. If it was easy, there would be no control-top industry, but that is the short answer. Strive to get over it and at least learn to navigate around it. Either way, don't use a distant goal as an excuse to put off enjoying or sharing your body. Be proud of your body, share it with zest, and you'll only add to your attractiveness. Remember, it's what you put behind it.

NAVIGATIONAL TIPS FROM WOMEN

Unfortunately, when it comes to dealing with negative body image there are far more things we can tell men not to do than to do.

- Don't make your devotion contingent on her appearance.
- Don't bring up her former great looks or point out how great other women look.
- Don't criticize her body in the name of "openness." Women's bodies are sort of like freaky relatives. We can rip them to shreds ourselves, but nobody else can.

Men need to tread very lightly and wisely in iceberg territory. Here is some guidance to men from women on how to proceed:

"No matter how logical a solution it may seem, don't suggest she lose weight or start exercising. *If she does decide to lose weight, let her come to that decision by herself for herself, then support her in every way. My husband got me a makeover and a gym membership for Christmas. I never asked for it and I was so hurt by that."*

"Give your wife the time she needs to reclaim a bit of herself. *When she gets some breathing space, chances are she will want to use that time to do something that makes her feel good."*

"Never comment on how much a woman is eating. *Healthy women eat in a healthy way and don't/shouldn't have to think about it all the time. Eat a lot together and appreciate meals."*

"When a woman makes fun of her body, do not fall into her trap and chime in. *She is merely trying to go there first to head off outside criticism at the pass."*

"It is important for a man to comment on what he does like about a woman's body *rather than the things that could be improved, such as: "I like those pants on you . . . You look really snazzy in that blouse . . . Those undies do something for me . . ."*

"When my husband touches me on the arm, waist, or anywhere non-sexual—especially in public, in broad daylight, and when I am fully clothed—*it makes me feel like he appreciates my body even when it doesn't have to do with sex. This simple gesture sends the message that he wants to caress me, not just my naked self, and because it is not an immediate sexual advance, it reassures my occasionally wobbly body image."*

"It helps when men acknowledge their own bodily genetic flaws and embrace them openly with good humor around women. *Somehow knowing men can accept their own imperfections helps women believe that men are more understanding of their physical imperfections."*

"**Tell women they are beautiful,** *even when they are dirty and sweaty.*"

"**Be naked together.** *Naked bodies should be shared and appreciated in the light and the dark. Love your mate's idiosyncrasies; whether it is a mole, love handles, and hefty hips . . . we all are beautifully imperfect.*"

"**Attach the word beautiful to all aspects of your mate,** *not just looks. Reinforce all the things she is and does that make her beautiful to you.*"

"**Celebrate the 'doing body' and don't worry so much about the 'looking body.'** *Help us to remember all the things our body does that enhance and give our lives meaning.* Sports Illustrated *may not be knocking on my door for their next swimsuit photo shoot, but I can walk my dogs until they are exhausted and happy. I mow, weed, put in flower beds, and haul yards of mulch so that I can step back and enjoy and take pride in my yard. These are real things that make me feel good and my body allows me to accomplish them. My husband can remind me of this the next time I point out something I don't like about my body.*"

"**Compliments are nice but they are tough because if the woman does not feel great about herself, then the compliment lies flat.** *What is better is when he invites me to do athletic activity with him. If we are truly engaged and happy, then our self-image will reflect that.*"

"**I have always (especially when naked) been self-conscious and disgusted about my butt.** *How can someone who is as active as I am still have cellulite? My husband responds along the lines of evolution and survival when I bring it up and somehow it makes me feel better.*"

"**Guys need to understand that for whatever reason we put WAY too much emphasis on how we are supposed to look** *and not on how important it is to feel good about ourselves. The toxic guys we may have met along our way have screwed us up by how they think we should look. Of course, it is important to take care of yourself and be healthy, but just because you have a few extra pounds on does not change who you are inside. Convincing ourselves of this is where we need guys to help us.*"

"**If men avoid openly checking out other women** *and their bodies, it will help their partners feel good about their bodies.*"

"**Occasionally, I would like to know that I look good from my husband's perspective.** *It would be great to have a little verbal validation.*"

"**No comments from the peanut gallery!** *If it is not going to make me feel good about my body don't say it. Do feel free to counteract your wife's comments about her areas of concern with endearing comments such as, 'I like your wrinkly belly because it makes me think of our two great kids.' or 'I love your strong legs . . . they turn me on.'*"

♀ ♂

"I hate the diaphragm. Trying to squeeze that frisbee in, with all that nasty goo, kind of kills the moment. The alternative—putting it in well ahead of time and have spermicidal gel dripping out of you—is even worse."
—female, age 42

"Vasectomies are fine—as long as they come with a guaranteed minimum of future nookie. This procedure is unilateral disarmament ("I'm turnin' in my bullets to the sheriff"). You have to get that nookie deal up front and in writing while you have still got the leverage (and the fire power)."
—male, age 39

Mirth Control: Contraception Is a Laughing Matter

The conception of a baby is a miracle. Preventing conception of a baby can feel like a miraculous feat. Sadly, a common feature afflicting so many of the available birth-control methods out there is that they can be a hassle to use and a deterrent to having sex. The effort and energy it requires to rig up the gear is often enough to squelch desire. Furthermore, the underlying issues related to birth control—who bears the responsibility for it, anxiety over effectiveness, resentment for the discomfort or possible side effects of certain kinds of birth control—are the types of slow-burning irritants that can fester into full-blown bitterness within a relationship. As always, bitterness and its close pal, resentment, lead us down the path to less sex, or at least less good sex. Still, birth control for most couples is a must and we are lucky to have choices. Our task is to find the ones that mesh with our lifestyles, our bodies, and our individual preferences.

HANDS-FREE VS HANDS-ON

Birth control options can be split into two categories: above-the-belt chemical options and below-the-belt physical barriers, some that release low doses of hormones. The above-the-belt options are clean and clinical—the pill, Depo-Provera shot, and Implanon (the successor of Norplant). At first, these inventions seemed like they solved the birth control issue, or at the very least, took the issue of birth control out of the relationship sphere. The birth control pill is the most widely used and effective form of birth control. Considering that the dosage of hormones and side effects have been greatly minimized, there appears to be no trade-off for the women who take this on.

But many women (and the men they live with) can tell you this science comes with a price. Hormonal fluctuations are challenging enough on their own that some women would prefer not to play with fire, either in the short term or the long term. Says one nurse and mother: "I hate the birth control methods available. Women's bodies are so complicated and once we start chemically messing with the reproductive system, we can get ourselves in trouble. It takes a few months to figure out if one is working or not, and when it's not working, you're not sure if it's your birth control or if you have cancer. When you finally figure out what works, you have kids or turn 40 and the whole thing changes!" Because all above-the-belt options can have side effects—some known and some possibly as yet undiscovered—some women don't want to mess with their body chemistry and are therefore limited to the hormone-free barrier options.

"I love condoms. It is one less mess I have to clean up and I actually find it a huge turn-on watching him put it on and then watching him rub his penis to keep his erection while he is putting it on!" —female, age 44

This is where it gets down and dirty and dicey—and quite a bit more hands-on. The most common choice is the condom, the Ford truck of contraception. Of course, you can get the Lamborghini and Ferrari versions with different colors, flavors, ribs, and ticklers, but flesh tones are the most convenient and accessible. While some couples complain about the decrease in sensitivity when using a condom, plenty of couples find it the no-muss, no-fuss solution. There is always the risk of breaking a condom, but even its failure is straightforward so you know immediately if and when to worry. In this situation, emergency contraception, sold as Plan B, can serve as safe effective backup,

> "With a husband on SSRIs (depression meds), famed for their negative effects in the bedroom, we needed enhanced sensation, and condoms were not an option. In the months of adjustment to the drugs, the last thing he needed was to enter into the male-castration-potential-dysfunction of anything in that murky zone. The fastest and safest by far was for me to step up. I took one for the team by getting an IUD." —female, age 41

especially when used within three days. It is not recommended to replace a regular form of birth control.

The intrauterine device (IUD) is an out-of-sight, out-of-mind kind of deal. When first introduced, they came in some interesting forms—the copper swirl, the question mark, or the thing that looks like it is made to scramble eggs. The two forms currently available in the United States are the Mirena and the Paraguard. After insertion, two arms spring up to make a capital T that resembles Jesus on the cross—a traffic cop for pesky, unwanted sperm. The Mirena acts as a barrier and releases low doses of a progestin hormone. The Paraguard provides a barrier without hormones, and releases copper to make sperm inactive. While the IUD seems to be gaining in popularity now that the infection and embedding issues have been largely remedied, some women still do find that the Paraguard puts them on the bench a couple of days each month. Overall the IUD option gives total freedom with maximum sensation. It is a draw, especially for women whose partners are taking any sort of medication that tweaks erectile dysfunction.

The newest insertion method, the NuvaRing (aka The Ring), is rising in popularity. It is a flexible, transparent vaginal ring two inches in diameter that releases a continuous low dose of estrogen and projestin. Reports from the trenches say it works well without noticeable side effects, but it does require being comfortable enough with your body to insert and remove it every three weeks.

Lest you think all these methods sound daunting and invasive, consider what many women went through when the diaphragm was in its heyday. The old trampoline is still an option for the brave and the tactilely adventureous. The man is not usually privy to diaphragm insertion, which is best categorized as an event, because he is in bed dutifully trying to maintain an erection. For the enlightenment of all men, this is what goes on while you are holding down (or rather holding up) the fort. The woman scurries to the bathroom, quickly unwraps her latex mini-tramp, and decorates the disk's outside ring and inner cup with spermicide goo. Truly, one needs an hour of yoga before trying to insert a diaphragm, but company is waiting at attention in bed, so even the Warrior Pose is out of the question at that point in the game. As she carefully folds and squeezes the slimy, gel-covered thing in preparation of cramming it into its tight parking spot, the diaphragm suddenly zings out of her hand and flies across the room like a liberated Frisbee in the park. These suckers can fly, so by the time you retrieve it you most likely have to blow off the dog hair before reloading. One woman's diaphragm was so crafty that it sailed right through the hole where the bathroom door's knob was supposed to be.

Once inside, the trampoline pops back into shape, all the while reefing on the walls of the vagina until finally it slurps into place around the cervix. You're not done until you ream your fingers around Up There to be sure it is in place. If your partner has managed to maintain an erection through all that, you get to have sex, but only once. No double dipping unless you take another Time Out with a small turkey baster–like rig to squirt a dose of sperm-killer goop back in there for Round Two. This routine helps explain why the diaphragm is also known as the Conception Accelerator.

> "The only good part about the diaphragm is that my daughter was conceived while using it!! I was conceived when my mom was using a diaphragm, so I guess it's a legacy."
> —female, age 43

In general, the responsibility for a particular form of birth control falls exclusively to either the man or the woman—with the man taking charge of and tolerating the effects of reduced sensitivity in condom territory, and the woman taking charge of and enduring the effects (mood swings, pulled muscles, blood loss) of all the other options. Rare is the opportunity for sharing the burden. The one exception is the female condom, an equal-opportunity inconvenience that takes the hands-on factor up one notch further. The concept of condoms made for women is empowering, and it reflects creativity on the part of our pharmaceutical and scientific community. Ideally, both partners should share the responsibility of contraception, but as Cindy's first and last experience with the method demonstrates (see What Do *We* Know?), it is unrealistic to expect such an interactive contraption to sweep a nation of largely uncommunicative sex partners. The female condom doesn't dominate the birth control section at pharmacies, but, ironically, it may be the best form of birth control because no man is going to want to have sex with a woman wrapped up in the female condom, unless he is turned on by mounting up on a Hefty garbage bag.

WHAT DO *WE* KNOW?

Cindy: "The windsock-like female condom has two rings—an outer ring and a floating ring that act like a diaphragm with a skirt once in place. The one time I tried it, insertion was like the diaphragm cram fest but when I stood up with the rig in place, it hung halfway to my knees, swinging like the Liberty Bell. I recovered from the shock of discovering that I had an exceptionally short vagina, and regained focus enough to begin my steamy walk to the bed. 'Fwap fwap fwap' it went as it swung against my inner thighs. My husband and I both realized that this would not be one of the sessions where the stars aligned, the skies opened up, and we were transported to some other dimension. This would be a science experiment. Usually lubrication is provided by the woman, but with the female condom hanging to my knees, artificial lubrication was required. Fortunately, they send a tube of the stuff along with the condom. We put in a squirt and gave it a go. The lube ran out quickly. Another squirt and gave it a go until it got squeaky. My husband decided he should just hold the lube tube for the sake of continuity. Squirt, squirt, squirt—another go. I started to laugh, 'I feel like the Tin Man with you and your oil can.' He was not amused, 'Stay focused, stay focused!' Needless to say, I got very little out of that session, and my husband, though he managed some semblance of closure to the event, admitted he felt like 'the boy in the plastic bubble.'"

Edie: "Most of my young adult life I used oral contraception, as in, 'Just say no.' Given my limited number of shots on goal combined with a reproductive system that conveniently went dormant with the stress of athletic competition, birth control never dominated my thoughts. I certainly never mastered it, and in fact one of my greatest blessings was a product of the Conception Accelerator (the diaphragm). Apparently I missed one or more of the seven steps of highly effective diaphragm use."

THE PERMANENT SOLUTION

These are but a few obstacles to birth control, and proof that an otherwise unspoken necessity can be an excellent source of humor. Of course the humor dissipates entirely when the method of choice fails. Condoms break, pills get forgotten, and IUDs make some women flow like Bloody Marys at a funeral. Bearing the bulk of both the physical and emotional strain of an unwanted pregnancy inspires women to be heavily invested in contraception, but when a couple has decided they don't want more (or any) children, the burden shifts back to the center. Any man who has experienced the heart-stopping effect of, "Honey, I'm a week late," knows the stakes. You're in it together and you are responsible for asking the questions and knowing the issues.

Given the inconvenient, uncomfortable, and uncertain nature of many forms of birth control, it's not surprising that many couples opt for the permanent birth control solutions. If your anxiety level about pregnancy has you using avoidance as a back-up form of birth control, you are a good candidate for one of these procedures.

> *"I may be one of the few woman against vasectomies. We have a thing against permanent prevention. I am not sure that there is enough info out there in the medical world. I wonder how a vasectomy affects mens' systems as they age."*
> —female, age 40

Sometimes there are clear health reasons to preserve one partner's fertility and not the other. If the woman happens to be having her fifth baby by C-section, then it's an easy choice to go tubal ligation. Essure, a device implanted into the fallopian tubes without incision or general anesthesia, offers women a non-surgical alternative for permanent birth control. Often women are just plain tired, not only of dealing with the birth control, but of tampering with their baby-making zones.

We've heard some really creative and desperate reasons that men have used to avoid vasectomies, like: "But honey . . . what if you betray me, take my kids, and I have to go out and re-create my family unit from scratch?" Or the ego-stoking "What if I'm the last fertile guy on earth?" One particularly reticent candidate merely stated, "I don't want to get my balls chopped off."

That is not how it works, of course. Technically, a vasectomy is quite straightforward. The doctor, after applying ample anesthetic, makes a slit in the scrotum and isolates a small section of the vas deferens, the tube that carries sperm from the manufacturing plant to the river of semen. With two clamps about an inch apart, the doctor snips a piece of the vas deferens out of its midsection. Both ends are sealed off with a staple or two, ensuring (usually) that they don't find each other and grow back together. That extremely rare and unfortunate reunion can happen and, on occasion, pesky sperm stage their own version of The Amazing Journey despite the fact that each end is cauterized for good measure.

Granted, the sight of smoke rising from Down There is undoubtedly unsettling, and sitting around with a bag of frozen peas on your crotch the next day isn't the ideal way to spend a Saturday. But trust us, we've seen some of the biggest skeptics admit it wasn't that bad. The most compelling endorsement for vasectomy comes from the doctor who spent a few weeks with "a nut the size of a softball and the color of an eggplant" and is still a vasectomy proponent.

We have yet to meet the man who has raised his hand and said, "I want a vasectomy," then used that same hand to actually pick up the phone in a timely manner. They may agree to it in theory, and even plan on it, but as far as actually making the appointment, that is rarely the voluntary action that, say, buying a new TV is. This is sacred territory for men, so women need to be patient and understanding . . . to a point. If your hints aren't working, make the appointment yourself. As best you can, screen the tales passed along to your partner. Anyone who makes reference to "balls swelling up to the size of grapefruits" should not be welcome in your home for the near term. One woman described the slow road to vasectomy, even after her husband decided to have one: "After two big scares, where I was two weeks late for my period, my husband realized he didn't want the stress and was going to have a vasectomy. A year later it hadn't happened, so I hinted. I spread the paper over his breakfast place to the article about vasectomies, left the phone book open to 'Urologists,' relayed every success story while casually dropping every reference I could to unplanned late-in-life pregnancies. Still, no appointment or commitment. Then he went to a college reunion and all his buddies (with no encouragement from me) pulled him aside and said how much it had changed their sex lives for the better. He finally picked up the phone."

THE SUNNY SIDE OF THE SNIP

Regardless of their universal reluctance, many men become big proponents of vasectomy once they are through it. One strong, silent type who never talks about intimate details admits, "It's not uncommon for me to go on vasectomy crusades now." An upside is that you are required to go on an ejaculation mission after the snip. Considering that you have endangered your manhood for the sake of the relationship, and that after the first week, you are under doctor's orders to "release the hostages" often, you likely will get a good spell of action. Having sex 15 times in two weeks is a tall order for anyone, let alone a married couple with kids, so don't expect quite that bonanza. Be creative with your leverage though, like the man who struck this bargain with his wife: "We made a deal. I do half and she does half." Another father of two said, "I was too embarrassed to wait for us to have sex that many times before I brought in my sample, plus I was eager to fly without a ticket, so I took matters into my own hands . . . a lot."

When you test clean, of course, you will have a freedom you've not known since before shaving. It's important to have a serious team huddle on any permanent solution because the guilt potential is not the kind of burden one partner should have to carry. You can try to get vasectomies reversed and tubes untied but there's no guarantee the ammo and the egg factories can be reactivated.

BOTTOM LINE

Birth control is a shared responsibility. Treat it as such and it can bring you closer by freeing up your sex life. Lay it all on one partner and it can drive a wedge between you.

WHY YOU SHOULD CARE

Cheaper by the Dozen was a really funny book and movie, but it was a work of fiction. Nothing pegs the stress meter like the prospect of an unwanted pregnancy.

WHAT YOU CAN DO

Even if one partner has always been the one to "deal with" birth control, make it part of community property in your relationship. Beyond the obvious benefit of finding the best birth control for you both, it demonstrates your willingness to share responsibility for a critical decision. Also, it is an effective vehicle for talking about your health issues, family plans, and of course your sex life—all things worth hashing out with each other.

"I discovered masturbation as a kid. I used to try to hold back and pace myself. Somehow I got the idea that you only got a certain number of orgasms rationed to you for life, and I didn't want to run out too soon."
—female, age 50

"Years ago after watching Fast Times at Ridgemont High, *one of the girls (she was hot) said, 'how about that guy jerking off?' and made a gesture. I didn't even know what jerking off was, but I went home and tried what she was doing. No lube or anything. I yanked on that thing. I almost pulled it out at the root. Finally, it exploded and scared me so much I swore I'd never do that again. I was back at it 15 minutes later."* —male age, 41

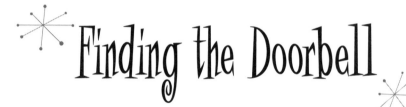

Finding the Doorbell

Your sexuality is just as much a part of your genetic code as your eye color and your temperament. The sooner you discover it, the sooner you can embrace and incorporate it into the rest of the unique package that is you. Alternatively, not "finding the doorbell" and exploring what lies beyond it can leave you feeling like you're on the outside looking into the colorful living room of the sexually awakened. Nobody wants to be on the outside looking in, especially at a really good party. Sexual pleasure is not something you find once and for all. Our bodies change constantly, in linear, cyclical, and just plain random ways. Both partners need to understand that finding the doorbell can be a new challenge every time and be willing to keep moving forward on the winding path to pleasure.

GETTING FROM CURB TO DOOR

As much as orgasm is a natural occurrence, it is a process for which we are usually unprepared and uneducated. This is especially true for women, largely because their own treasures are literally hidden beneath the mysterious waves and layers of the vulva. While boys can compare their gear in the locker room and watch how it responds to various stimuli, girls are left to their own assumptions on how to have an orgasm or even what it feels like. Socially and culturally we are taught from an early age not to touch ourselves Down There, not to talk about it if we do, and certainly not to expect congratulations for our discovery. Guilt or secrecy associated with early sexual experiences, if left unaddressed, can be parasitic anxiety that quietly adheres to our adult sex lives and makes us feel guilty about sexual pleasure. Thanks to that cloak of secrecy and shame, "Finding the Doorbell" is a complex challenge, first for girls and later for the men who want to please them.

WHAT DO *WE* KNOW?

Cindy: "The few women who openly talked about orgasms during high school and college led me to believe all sexually active women were having orgasmic sex, and since I was righteously holding onto my virginity until I felt mutual love, I had no reason to doubt that.

"My first physical encounters with trusted guy friends were positive and healthy, filled with open discussion, partially clothed exploration, honesty, and humor. Good sensations but no Big O. Then, in my senior year in high school, a good friend gave me a reality check: 'You gotta get on it yourself before you can expect the guys to know how to do it.' In deference to my Catholic influences she offered a hands-free technique. 'Get yourself in the bathtub, put the faucet on a slow drip, saddle your hips under there and let it drip on the top of your vagina.' Initially, I was horrified, but her enticing description of orgasms inspired me to get over it and get in the tub. It was a very efficient way to get things moving, and if I had not been so attention-challenged, I may have made it to the Promised Land. No such luck.

"In college, another friend encouraged me to quit soccer and join the bike team. 'I ride behind hot guys in Lycra with my bike seat angled in such a way that I'm kicking out miles of orgasms.' I wasn't convinced enough to buy a bike. My graphic sister Winston described an orgasm, by prattling on about the build-up of intensity with feet shaking and body quaking, ending with a volcanic eruption. Her description convinced me that I was either adopted or that she was blessed with super, turbo-charged gear while I had been cursed with a little putt-putt.

"Finally, I discovered mutual love that led to sex, and I was ready to blast off for the real deal. Sexual intercourse certainly brought the arousal level up significantly, but it was more like that dog-itch thing—that pesky itch that can't be relieved. I wasn't getting over the top. I had made it through the desert only to find more mountains to climb. My panel of wise women and my boyfriend assured me that the position of one's clitoris determines whether intercourse alone will bring you around the bend. I learned most women require his hand, a vibrator, or her own hand in the mix. Practice, different positions, and exploration are also needed to find the best way to bring a woman to climax. With my boyfriend living all the way across the country I didn't have much time to practice.

"And then one night . . . I went to the library the night after my boyfriend headed back home. Being sequestered to a carrel to maximize my focus and productivity didn't deter me from thinking about sex, this new and exciting part of my life. After my thoughts drifted there one too many times, I took a bathroom break to help me refocus. While wiping myself, I ran smack dab into my clitoris. Something about all those steamy thoughts had worked me into a lather, and my clitoris presented itself front and center, practically begging my hand to come around front and check it out. Within moments, I had such a whopper of an orgasm, I nearly fell off the toilet and cracked my head on the tile floor.

"After pulling myself together I cleaned up and hustled back to my carrel, feeling like everyone in the library would see my flushed cheeks and satisfied grin, and know what I had been up to. Five minutes later I was back in the bathroom giving myself the business again."

Edie: "Chalk one up for the Puritan, I never had a problem getting off and for all I knew nobody else did either. It seemed pretty simple. You have a little friction with a guy you like, you have an orgasm. It is only in retrospect that I feel a bit guilty for going along my merry way satisfied with those clothed encounters, and leaving virtually every guy high and dry. Maybe I never learned to talk about it because I never had to. At any rate, being easily entertained left me with one less symptom of repression."

FLYING SOLO

As it turns out, women having their first orgasms by themselves and by mistake is not that unusual. Although orgasms are associated with sex, they can happen well before it's appropriate to even have the language to discuss it, let alone the opportunity. Many women can't remember their first orgasm because they started masturbating so young that it was an incentive to get out of diapers. Certainly by grade school it's already open season for many girls. A second-grade teacher recalls feeling a pang of remorse at seeing one of her students nearly collapse in rapture and realizing a seven-year-old was more sexually fulfilled than she was. Even for less exploratory youths, or those whose parents terrified them from ever exploring the land down under, there are all manner of childhood activities that seem designed to awaken us. C'mon, what girl can ride a horse without scootching around in the saddle a bit? Why did climbing the ropes in gym have such appeal? How about the pool jet? Skiers, can we talk about the Poma lift? That little razzle dazzle, even if it didn't get you over the top, certainly was enough to inspire curiosity.

Some girls (a lot more than you'd suspect), got busy with anything soft and portable, like pillows, twisted blankets or sheets, and especially, their stuffed animals. Because shame and guilt hinder such powerful sensation from leading to meaningful discussion, early orgasm experiences tend to build into a much greater mystery for some of us. Depending on your outlets for processing complex feelings at that young age, these memories can carry all the fixins' for either lifelong therapy or lifelong humor. For many, the biggest fear in these early explorations was getting caught. One woman recalls the panic of seeing her father innocently waving at her through her bedroom window from his lawn tractor while she was getting busy with her stuffie.

> *"I had my first orgasm touching myself in fourth grade. I was panicked and was convinced I was pregnant. It just seemed so momentous, how could it not cause something like a baby."* —female, age 42

SO THAT'S WHAT IT IS

While some lucky girls get counsel from friends and sisters, many rely on whatever sources and situations present themselves. One woman first learned about orgasms while reading *The Color Purple* where Sophie talks about her "button." Others just get lucky with the company they keep. One woman describes how she was fooling around with her boyfriend in high school, "and suddenly he hit a spot I did not realize I even had. Yahoo!" A man recalls feeling around with his fingers on a girlfriend in high school and then hitting the buzzer: "I knew she had an orgasm because her whole body tensed up, and she farted."

Some women are simply born with good alignment, so that their clitoris is positioned for direct response more similar to the progression of the male orgasm. For these women, orgasms usually precede their first actual sexual experiences because there's no telling what source of stimulation will scratch the itch once the clitoris is aroused. One woman was "totally freaked out" by an orgasm while putting in her first tampon at age 16. Another woman's first orgasm ambushed her when her young lover seated her on a running dryer. You had to know there was a trade-off to the convenience of stackable appliances. In case you have ever wondered about the power of the mind in basic sexual response, consider the women whose first orgasms came without any kind of stimulation, while she was lying on a rock in the sun halfway up a mountain. "I didn't even put it together and figure out what it was until later. I guess I've always been a nature girl."

Boys have far less ambiguity when it comes to orgasms. While girls privately seek or try to comprehend the capricious and elusive orgasm, boys seem to have an explosive and virtually transparent discovery. While some men remember getting the full sensation of their first orgasm while shooting a blank, most others recall there was no hiding the proof. Perhaps because of the tangible residual evidence, boys' reactions to orgasms are typically more triumphant or at least more open than the girls' experiences. One man remembers playing with his penis regularly as a boy and making it hard, liking the effect but thinking it was not very satisfying. Then he awoke one night in the throws of massive orgasm resulting from his first wet dream. "AWESOME! I was hooked!" Another clearly recalls the night before Christmas when he was 11 years old. "I told my younger brother on the lower bunk, 'Dude, some crazy shit just happened.'"

> "I was on my bike, gaining speed down a bumpy road, with my junk resting on the seat and rattling away. It stopped me dead in my tracks. I must have ridden it 100 more times down that same road hoping, hoping, but I never got it that way again." —male, age 48

DRUMROLL PLEASE

From the stories we heard, first encounters with intercourse were all over the map: good or bad, painful or uneventful, harmless or scarring, powerful or pathetic. Each of us has our unique story. Chances are it was not the extreme you expected, but that's what you take as a first impression for the rest of your life. The hope is that we can use those first experiences—that were often so built up that the reality felt like a step backward—as a benchmark for how much better sex gets. For those of us who blithely assumed orgasms and sex went together like milk and cookies, the journey had just begun.

One woman remembers trying really hard to have an orgasm on her own: "It just didn't work. Then I lost my virginity—30 seconds of massive pain with a guy with a huge penis—I couldn't believe that's what sex was."

Orgasms coinciding with starter sex are so rare, that many young sexually active women don't look toward their sexual futures with much optimism. Girls and women who have already experienced orgasms before having intercourse have nonetheless built up "real sex" in their minds, and often react to the typical fast, nervous first experience with, "That was it?"

"It" is not typically explained to girls by anyone and, because the whole pleasure zone is hidden, they are usually on their own in even figuring out what an orgasm feels like. One woman had to use deductive reasoning to recognize her first orgasm, which happened to be during sex: "The only way I knew I was having one was because I was moaning and starting to sound like women do in the movies and on TV."

BOTTOM LINE

Finding the doorbell is a specific achievement or moment, but the terminology represents much more. It is the mechanism for getting in touch with ourselves, to opening the door for our way to please ourselves and ultimately our partners.

WHY YOU SHOULD CARE

Couples need sex, and if they want it to be mutually satisfying, they need orgasms. Men want to give women orgasms, but they often can't figure it out without women's help. It is up to the women to understand their bodies and explain what they've learned to men. It is up to men to be open to, and solicitous of, that direction.

> "I spent a long time wondering if I was incapable of having an orgasm. I think a lot of women have a hard time figuring out their own bodies, and I think there are so many reasons for this. I felt that I was never trained or taught to think about my own needs while having sex. I was also so self-conscious about my body that I wasn't even present. It was like watching myself have sex instead of actually having it."
> —female, age 34

WHAT YOU CAN DO

Cindy's library moment inspired her mission and her motto to GET ON IT! When guys lined up to feast on her every tidbit of information when she had a grand total of two orgasms under her belt, she realized the truth: For all their rummaging around vaginas, men don't necessarily know where the goodies reside. They feel like they are groping around, searching for the prize in the bottom of the Cracker Jack box. Sometimes they come up with it, and sometimes they don't. The first step is to understand your own body and its needs. The next step is to discover your partner's needs. Exchanging your stories is a good place to start—whether it's sordid or funny or beautiful or embarrassing, you are not alone. Orgasms, like the hokey pokey, are what it's all about, so read on and take the motto to heart: GET ON IT!

Section II:
What's the Big O Deal?

by Edie Thys Morgan

While Cindy was on her mission of orgasm research and education, I, as a dutiful member of the Silent Majority, paid no attention whatever to the phenomenon. In fact, the Silent Majority had a good long run of keeping down orgasm chat until 1948, when the zoologist Alfred Kinsey came out with his groundbreaking study called *Sexual Behavior in the Human Male* and five years later its sequel, *Sexual Behavior in the Human Female*. Based on extensive surveys with over 10,000 men and women, Kinsey's reports revealed that people indeed had sex for reasons other than procreation. In fact they had a lot of it, together, alone, and in all manner of combinations that were not previously considered proper conversation. Kinsey's research, while socially shocking, opened the door for the work of William Masters and Virginia Johnson, whose pioneering book, *Human Sexual Response*, was released in 1966. Whereas Kinsey's method of extensive face-to-face surveys took the field mouse approach, Masters' and Johnson's work relied on the lab rat methodology, rigging 700 subjects with polygraph-like devices to measure sexual response. Their research identified the four phases of the human sexual response cycle—excitement, plateau, orgasm, and resolution—the orgasm template for all subsequent physiological sex studies.

Kinsey cracked the repressive seal of secrecy around sex so that Masters and Johnson could blow open the conversation on orgasms. Both, however, failed to fully address how the sexual response cycle differs between men and women. The conclusions didn't take into account the physiological differences in arousal between males and females, or the non-physiological influences on orgasm, both of which are significant. Society had a lot more information, but not a clear understanding of why the male and female sexual experience is so different and how we might help each other make it better. More recent studies support that normal female sexual response is a circular, feedback-based process rather than a linear process. Female arousal incorporates sexual stimuli as well as non-physical factors such as emotional intimacy and relationship satisfaction.

Any conversation about orgasm has the potential to be awkward, but it can get even more so when talking to people in long-term relationships. Orgasm is all about sensation, and the more invested we become in other aspects of our relationship the more reluctant we are to talk about our selfish pursuits of pure pleasure. We tend to talk about how we think we should feel sexually instead of how we do feel sexually. This is especially true of men in long-term relationships, especially those with kids, who feel bitter about not getting enough sexual satisfaction or guilty about wanting more pleasure. For that reason we reached out to the young bucks to round out the discussion about orgasm in this section. These men in their early 20s, who we call Pre-Bitterness and Guilt—PBG—males, offered their un-edited wish lists with no threat of repercussion from potentially surly or dissatisfied women.

The topic of female orgasm is thornier, because few women even know what leads them to orgasm, let alone how to articulate it. Years ago, someone told me about attending a masturbation workshop led by a self-described orgasm doctor in New York. I listened with compassion, because I knew her sex life had been severely challenged by a date rape in her youth. I did not, however, remotely imagine the day I would come face to face with the maven of masturbation: a woman whose books, videos, and private sessions have led countless women to discover comfort with their own bodies and their orgasmic potential; a woman who commands $1,100 for one session that can last hours; a woman who can offer a Consumer Reports–like analysis of vibrators. Betty Dodson is a 77-year-old artist, author, and sexologist who agreed to meet with us in her New York apartment to share her encyclopedic knowledge of the female orgasm.

Dodson recoils from any form of euphemism. She insists on saying CLIToris rather than cliTORis, because that's the way it would be phonetically, and she doesn't believe in dressing up the language of sex in any way. As we romped through topics of orgasms and masturbation, vaginal mapping, sex toys, and more anatomy than I wanted to know, she enthralled us with her passion for it all.

Dodson adheres to a basic philosophy that, "The key to a woman being consistently orgasmic is when she gets to the age or place that she takes control of her own clitoris, when she can say, 'I am responsible for my own orgasm.' No woman is truly non-orgasmic. It's a lack of information." She espouses that having orgasms isn't about getting your man or learning to subject yourself for someone else's pleasure. It is about taking command of your own flight. You have to put your own oxygen mask on before you can help others.

Before meeting Dodson I feared she would find us hopelessly vanilla for her realm. She did. Nonetheless she gently suggested ways to enliven our aspirations and when we pressed her on any hope she could offer to monogamous couples she put her head in her hands on the table and groaned, "You people!" But then she rallied with a list of recommendations for monogamy that we share in Section III, Sex for the Long Haul. Even while she is appalled that we don't use sex toys, she agrees with us on the end result of their purpose. "Even if you get one and use it twice and it gets thrown out it's worth it. Anything that sets progress in motion—even if it's just a conversation—is a good thing. All anyone can ask for is that couples talk more."

Leaving her apartment, full of enlightening information I didn't know I was missing, I recalled crying at the end of Kinsey the movie, thinking of all the people who suffered from not being able to talk about sex before he broke the ice. Having come in filled with dread, I left filled with gratitude for the good doctor. We owe all the Dr. Orgasms though the ages an enormous debt. Because of them the Big O Deal—what it is, why we want it, and how we get it—is no secret.

The Inside Dope

O f course, we know you know, and that you know we knew it already, but just in case we all need a refresher, what, exactly, is an orgasm? With guys, thanks to their well-displayed plumbing, it's pretty obvious, even if it is a complex interaction of bodily systems. Dr. Susan Bennett describes what she refers to as the point and shoot process: "Erection and ejaculation (orgasm) are separate physiological events. Erection is under the control of the parasympathetic (point) nerves and relies on a very healthy arterial supply. Ejaculation is under the control of the sympathetic (shoot) nerves and is not as dependent on vascular health."

THE JOURNEY BEGINS

Essentially, the man gets excited, blood flow surges to the penis, which (ideally) obediently and firmly salutes. From there, momentum typically sweeps the man down a preordained "lemmings to the sea" journey. With a token amount of sexual stimulation, excitement continues, the reflex centers of the spinal cord urge the genitals to call up their fluid providers to build up pressure in the urethra, then the groin muscles fire with contractions. Houston, we have lift-off. Within one to two minutes the penis goes back to rest as (often) does its keeper.

A woman's journey has the same itinerary—excitement, plateau, orgasm, and resolution—but her flight plan is a little more complicated, to say the least. Like the man's trip, hers starts with some sort of sexual stimulus, mental or physical. Her early phase looks similar: breathing, heart rate, and blood pressure accelerate; skin gets flushed and sweaty; pupils dilate;

key players—nipples and clitoris—become erect and exposed. Up to now she's on track with the guy. The only problem is that this phase can last 20 minutes or much more, while her pathway to pleasure ascends, plateaus, dips, and rolls, all the while deciding whether or not it's even going to lead her to the "point of inevitability" as psychologists call it. If she passes that point, orgasm is one big tension release delivered in a series of involuntary and thoroughly pleasurable muscular contractions, the grand finales of which last an average 13 seconds in duration. The body stiffens, the muscles contract, and spasms may occur from her legs and stomach to her arms and back. Her sensations can range from mildly pleasant to volcanic—to downright headscrambling as the muscles of the uterus and vagina relax and contract rapidly, while the body discharges lubricating fluid.

FLIGHT STIMULATORS

Sounds like the ultimate thrill, and it is, if you can hang in there long enough for an orgasm to happen. It all comes down to stimulation, and in the case of women, lots of it. Again, basic stimulation for the male is straightforward and focused on the "main man" standing tall. With women there are various stimulation sites, with command central being the button-like tip of the clitoris, which lends itself relatively easily to doting attentions with its quaking response to excitement. The runner-up for most stimulating player is the coy, elusive, controversial G-spot that can produce or enhance orgasms, along with all manner of erogenous zones, from nipples to earlobes. The G-spot's discoverer and namesake, Dr. Ernst Grafenberg, claimed that the spongy, grape-sized area lurks a couple of inches up inside the frontal wall of the vagina (see Orgasm Mechanics). If you think Dr. G had a good job, consider the daily grind for the "licensed sex surrogates," people whose job it is to cure non-orgasmic women. Seriously, they're out there.

But as is typical in the female orgasm discussion, we digress. Suffice it to say, there are a lot more variables that go into the women's process, and these are only the visible signs that we can manipulate. What we don't see in both male and female orgasm processes is even more compelling. Take it all into a lab and it turns out orgasms serve up a potent dose of dopamine, the neurochemical that activates the "reward center" of your brain, which is the part that drives nearly all of your behaviors. This center is activated when you engage in activities that generally further your survival or the continuation of your genes—things like procuring food, water, acceptance, and yes, sex. Behind all these "urges" lies the brain's craving for dopamine and its constant drive to receive that next "hit."

EVE GOT A BREAK

While male orgasm is necessary for procreation because semen is ejaculated by orgasm, there is no evidence that female orgasm is necessary for procreation. Women got lucky then, that the clitoris arises from the same embryologic organ as the penis and is thus a repository of erectile tissue. Susan Bennett concludes, "While no one knows for sure the exact proportion of women who have orgasms with intercourse, research suggests that less than 25 percent of women experience regular orgasm with penetrative sex. However, the vast majority of women can experience orgasm with adequate clitoral stimulation, which can be incorporated into the activity of intercourse."

This potentiality is the critical factor that keeps women motivated for sex because orgasms deliver a boatload of dopamine—some evidence suggests on par with heroine rushes. Dopamine fuels a self-perpetuating cycle where having orgasms makes you want more of them. This is good news for anyone angling for more sex and great news for anyone angling for better sex. This childhood melody about love could just as well be about orgasms:

It's just like a magic penny,
Hold it tight and you won't have many
Lend it spend it and you'll have so many
They'll roll all over the floor.

Rolling on the floor. Imagine that!

DOPAMINE JUNKIES

Of course, there is a downside. The vagaries of the dopamine reward system lie in the fact that when it comes to getting its "fix," the primal brain is not overly discriminating. It compels us to want sex, but has no qualms about who or what we have sex with and, in fact, reaffirms our primitive predisposition to find different partners and maximize survival of the species. Fortunately, we are among the 3 percent of mammals (in good company with prairie voles) designed for social monogamy, thanks to the cocktail of chemicals that accompany sex and orgasms. Among them oxytocin and vasopressin—the "cuddling" hormones—compel us to do silly, Darwinistically irresponsible things like fall in love and seek a more complete variety of happiness. If you care to read up on it, there are biological rationales not only for why we have sex and crave orgasms, but also for what motivates attraction for each gender, why we fall out of love, cheat, lose our sex drive, fall asleep after sex, and do all manner of unsociable things. But let's proceed on the assumption that we will strive to get beyond the primitive brain mechanisms here, and try to embrace the behaviors and physical processes that support our relationships in a healthy, mutually respectful way.

BOTTOM LINE

We are hard-wired not only to have orgasms but to want more of them. You're having them or you're not. You all know who you are.

WHY YOU SHOULD CARE

Orgasms, however much credit we give them, are an interaction of physical and emotional processes that are an evolutionary necessity. Hard science, as well as our own experiences, back up our desires, not only for sex but for good, satisfying, orgasmic sex. We believe knowing how it all really works can help you assess your toolbox, reorganize and update it if necessary, and make strides toward enhancing your sex life.

WHAT YOU CAN DO

Knowledge is power. The first step is getting to know your own body and how it responds to stimulation. Then try to learn, understand, respect, and meet the needs of your partner. Note that understanding the chemistry of sex and orgasms does not give you license to cheat. The overwhelming biological need to spread your seed, or leave your spouse because you are programmed to find the best provider is a caveman/cavewoman defense that holds no weight in twenty-first-century standards of decency. Sleeping around is just plain unacceptable. The payoff for monogamy—and there ought to be one—is that you have ample opportunity to get to explore and discover all the ways to bring each other pleasure.

♀ | ♂

"If we have an exceptionally orgasmic sex experience, he usually uses the same approach the next time we have sex. Unfortunately, my body doesn't always respond to the same kind of stimulus. If I want to have an orgasm, he explores while I give guidance until we find the way that it can happen." —female, age 35

"She put her hand over mine and directed my fingers on and around her clitoris. That was key. I was so pumped when she came. I could make it happen on my own after that." —male, age 28

✳ Orgasm Mechanics ✳

One bold and befuddled guy admitted, "It took me five years to get my girl's shit off. Pardon me, but five years." He went on to sum up his source of bewilderment. "How about the vagina with all the flaps and folds, it's like origami." He is not alone in bemoaning this challenge. Men and boys may differ wildly, but their gear is not complicated. For guys, having an orgasm is like swinging by the ATM. For women, it's like breaking into Fort Knox. Not only are the origami-like flaps and folds of the vulva mystifying, but the clitoris is moody. What works one day may not the next. Complicated as it can be, guys can take heart in the overwhelming evidence of what they're up against and the notion that bringing a woman to orgasm need NOT be the full responsibility of the man.

INFORMATION PLEASE

Finding a psychic partner, however convenient that would be, is highly unlikely, and yet that is what women expect when they say they want their guy just to know what they like. This is mean, considering the complicated nature of origami and the fact that this task requires patience, teamwork, and guidance. Many women won't speak up because they don't want to make a man feel inadequate, while men are reluctant to ask for guidance because they think they know or are supposed to know what to do. The following clues are not meant to bum you out guys, but to make men and women feel better if they have had any challenge giving or achieving orgasms.

THE FACTS

- Men take an average of four minutes or less to reach orgasm while women take an average of 20 minutes to climax.
- Less than 15 percent of women report being non-orgasmic. Betty Dodson (aka "Dr. Orgasm" for her 100 percent success rate at coaching women to orgasm) believes being non-orgasmic is a function of not having the right information.
- Male orgasms obey a predictable FMW formula—friction, moisture, and warmth—while there is no formula that guarantees a female orgasm.
- Many dildos and vibrators on the market have extensions to stimulate the clitoris while the phallus part penetrates the vagina.
- Condoms are available with vibrators at the base.
- A recent review of the sexology literature reports that less than 25 percent of women reach orgasm with intercourse alone. That leaves a whole lot of us in need of extra stimulus.
- Clitoral-mapping workshops exist and are well-attended. These are intended for women to help them get in touch with their orgasm potential.

Lack of communication lowers the odds of female orgasms significantly. One way or another, everyone needs guidance from a reliable source. One man told how a tip from a friend changed his life: "When I was 17, I asked my friend about giving orgasms because when I was looking for the clitoris, I felt like I was way up there trying to extract a booger. He said, 'No dude, it's the little man in the boat. Find it.' I found it!"

GOOD WITH THEIR HANDS

Even though the clitoris can be a pesky, elusive little bugger, men may find it helpful to approach giving a woman an orgasm as a mechanical pursuit. Some women, albeit a minority, are factory tuned with a clitoris that is lined up for direct contact during intercourse. Most, however, require that you get under the hood — exposing the clitoris by pulling up the labia— and get your hands, if not dirty, at least wet by using extra lube or saliva. Women need to be patient with their men who are trying to please them while maintaining their own staying power. It's not an easy feat, especially for young bucks like this 26-year-old who told us, "If my girlfriend tells me she is about to climax, I blow my load immediately. I can't help it."

Timing that stimulation to achieve orgasm while the penis is in the vagina adds a level of complexity to the task. The "bridge technique," which is essentially using your fingers to stimulate the clitoris and then inserting the penis at just the right time can be a bit like patting your head and rubbing your stomach—tough to coordinate at first, but you eventually get used to it. In theory at least, the brain receiving signals from an adequately stimulated clitoris eventually develops a Pavlovian response to the impending insertion of the penis—eagerly anticipating it because of its association with the stimulation.

Of course, we all would prefer to simply rely on nature taking care of the process, but one of nature's cruel little jokes is that men and women do not have coordinated sexual response cycles. (On the other hand, with age this difference in timing works out nicely because the guy can hang in there until the 20-to-40-minute effort pays off.)

Some women, in an effort to make their partners feel good, or simply to move the process along, fake orgasms. Tsk, tsk (see Faking It: The Inhumane Option). Men are mostly hurt and annoyed by this and would much rather help her achieve an orgasm. But they could sure use some guidance and participation. Reinforcing false confidence isn't helping anyone in the long run. Men need extraordinary patience to rummage around all the vagina's nooks and crannies, finding where the ignition lies, as well as the angle of the day that's going to kick it over.

FANCY FINGERWORK

"Some positions make it easier to access the clitoris, but the missionary position is the most intimate for my wife and me. I support myself with one hand or elbow and use one or two fingers to stimulate her clitoris while having intercourse." —male, age 44

"I use the thumb. It is definitely easier on the hand and I can go for longer because my wrist isn't in an unnatural position. If a woman tells me to go harder, I might push down a bit more with my thumb. It is mostly just circular motion to stimulate the clit. I have had phenomenal results with it . . . a credit to internet porn actually." —male, age 22

"I use the two-finger pitter-patter. Very effective." —male, age 40

G WHIZ: BEYOND THE BUTTON

Named after Dr. Ernest Grafenberg, the G-spot was first described by the good doctor in 1950 as the spongy (think rough sea sponge) tissue around the urethra opening two inches up on the front inside wall of the vagina. When not aroused, it is about the size of a pea and grows to lima bean stature when awoken. The G-spot is credited for heightened pleasure, deeper orgasms, and female ejaculation (also called squirting). Controversy arises because while many women attest to its power, others report having an undetectable or unresponsive G-spot, and some greet its stimulation with mild to moderate annoyance. Even the terminology is confusing, especially in reference to the G-"spot," which can be more of a zone for some women.

Orgasms emanate not only from the clitoris, but also from a variety of zones that vary with each woman, including the much-debated G-spot. There are erogenous zones all over the body that can contribute to an orgasm, but for the purpose of this G-spot primer, we are referring to the immediate V-zone (the area around the vulva and vagina). Most women agree that there are responsive spots or areas inside the vagina, which seem to deepen orgasms, and possibly cause squirting in some women. There is more going on in this zone alone than Air Traffic Control at O'Hare could handle. For many women, the most sensitive areas are unpredictable. The kicker du jour could be a specific spot on the side of the clitoris one day, in a random labial zone on another, and along the front wall of the vagina on yet another day—a moving target that changes camp more haphazardly than a band of gypsies. This gatekeeper, wherever it lays in wait for the keymaster on a particular day, adds to the pleasure but usually isn't the source of big-bang orgasms like the clitoris is for most women (see Gimme an O! Gimme Another O!).

Although we want to avoid encouraging men to bank their whole mission on finding the G-spot, enough rave reviews from women warrant liberating the G-spot from the witness-protection program. Here's the good news for explorers. Unlike the clitoris, which is easy to find yet finicky to please, the G-spot, once located, usually responds best to steady pressure.

We're not talking the demure doorbell press of a girl scout selling cookies. Think of pushing on the buzzer like a persistent bill collector. For some women this kind of consistent pressure results in female ejaculation and for a number of women pressure in this area deepens the clitoral orgasm. The available research is so inconclusive that some experts refer to it as the "so-called" G-spot. According to Betty Dodson in *The G-Spot Revisited* the most current research shows that what we've been calling the "G-spot" is connected with "a cluster of tiny prostate-like glands located inside a tube of spongy tissue surrounding the urethra that lies above the vaginal ceiling (paraurethral gland—which encompasses the vaginal wall two inches inside the vulva)." The idea of responsive spots spread out in the barrel of the vagina explains why women prefer a more varied medley of stimulation. Here is yet another compelling reason for women to give explicit direction and for men to solicit guidance.

The medical community is limited to available studies as well as reports from their patients. Few of the studies focus on exploring sexual potential beyond the context of sexual dysfunction. Furthermore, the doctor's office is not an environment conducive to uninhibited talk about sexual satisfaction. Even the most open, comfortable women we interviewed rarely engage their health professional in what they see as a private, non-medical matter. When it comes to maximizing sexual function, unconventional programs (such as clitoral mapping and masturbation workshops) that might not show up in the Yellow Pages are where the deeper secrets of orgasmic potential are unearthed and openly discussed.

While the prospect of distilling all of this physiological information into useful sexual knowledge seems overwhelming, remember—when it comes to creating satisfying orgasms, the clitoris reigns supreme. In most women, the clitoris is not in the line of penetration, and the most intense orgasms come from clitoral stimulation—with fingers, a thumb, or a vibrator—combined with penetration. This "blended orgasm," not to be confused with an umbrella drink, effectively accommodates virtually all anatomy.

HAND JOBS 101—ADVICE FROM THE PBG GUYS*

"I will stop a girl from giving me a dry hand job. I won't be mean about it, but if no lube is present I will just find some way to stop her. Girls tend to grip hard the whole time, creating lots of friction instead of squeezing on the way down and releasing more on the way up. They also just go straight up and down instead of in a more circular motion. Some girls go really hard and actually slam their hand on my balls at the very bottom and that is not the type of stimulation my boys need."
—male, age 22

"Some type of lubrication is a must, whether it is a combo of blow job/hand job or something else that isn't going to cause chafing or burn. More important is to know exactly the technique that each guy likes. Every guy enjoys something different. The majority of women just don't understand the concept of a handy. They are better off asking the guy what feels good or just not attempting it at all. When all else fails, men enjoy masturbating by themselves a lot more that receiving a bad handy." —male, age 21

"Dry hand jobs are horrible. You can get through it, but I can do a better job on my own. Lube is key for a hand job by a woman." —male, age 25

*young bucks in the Pre-Bitterness and Guilt stage of their lives

WHAT DO WE KNOW?

Cindy: "Orgasms are a random deal. My husband is the most enthusiastic, patient participant, ready to explore and navigate in any way to make it happen, but it can take a long time to get to the first orgasm (sometimes 30 minutes). Each time we have sex, it is a different combination of events that lead to a climax and the result is never predictable. It could require nipple stimulation along with penetration and clitoral stimulation with his finger. Other times I am tapped into various sensitive zones inside my vagina with different areas on fire at different times including clitoral stimulation. It is all about combinations with trial and error. It is quite a job for him to be so adaptable and focused, but he always shows up for work."

Edie: "Ah, the life of the innkeeper. I was intrigued and doubtful when I heard the G-spot referred to as 'knobby tissue,' so I decided to ramble around in there and check it out. It wasn't exactly knobby, but the texture was certainly unsettling for being tucked away as it is. Furthermore, feeling it was more annoying than anything, which makes me think I'll hold off on the G-spot quest until a later stage of life, when I hope to have time for all kind of things like weeding my garden, taking up golf, and perhaps running a country inn."

BOTTOM LINE

The source of orgasm is never consistent. Everyone has their zones and spots, and we suggest mapping them out on your own or with your trusted partner. Prepare to evolve day to day and over time.

WHY YOU SHOULD CARE

Women deny themselves orgasms for various reasons: they have never had one, feel overwhelmed by the time commitment, are uncomfortable with their bodies, don't feel they are deserving of the effort, or think a man's satisfaction is more important. The way we see it, orgasms are only as selfish as taking care of oneself with good nutrition, rest, laughter, and exercise. Furthermore, most men claim giving orgasms to women is such a boost that it's a major turn-on.

WHAT YOU CAN DO

Men: Spending time finding out just what she likes could really improve your experience. Don't be afraid to get your hands wet, and do remember to clip your nails. Let her take you through the motions—her hand over your hand—to learn what turns her on. Put your ego away and shamelessly open the door for guidance, because some women won't speak up for fear of hurting your feelings. You may be surprised how much help you receive. Ask, ask, ask, and convince her that you both benefit by having some way to communicate each other's needs. If she is critical of you for asking or doesn't respond, she is a fool, and an unlucky, no-action fool at that.

Women: If you invest a little more time in facilitating your own orgasms you could benefit greatly. Open your mind to extra clitoral stimulation from his finger or your own during intercourse. There are many mini-vibrators commonly used, readily camouflaged, and easily acquired to help clitoral stimulation during intercourse if less direct contact makes you more comfortable. Here's the rub—if you want to be pleased by others, you have to get in there and explore your own unique setup (see Taking Matters Into Your Own Hands.) Once you know yourself, the chances of your partner learning how to give you ultimate pleasure goes up tenfold. Speaking up could change your sex life. If you can't speak up, find some way to provide GPS-like guidance—like a subtle Ouija board nudge with your hand on his. Don't forget that enhancing the male orgasm, while it may not seem challenging, is absolutely possible. Mixing it up with hand jobs, oral sex, and different positions can heighten his experience. Most of all, be engaged and responsive.

♀ ♂

"Oral sex elicits a very surface sensation on the first orgasm. The second one, which happens soon after with intercourse, is much deeper and intense. I can't help making this sort of stifled scream that sounds like it comes from a different place in me."
—female, age 37

"Teasing makes an orgasm more intense. Teasing to the point of being cruel. Make me wait and wait and wait for the orgasm, bringing me close, take it away, bring me close again, take it away, over and over. Then, when the blast off finally arrives, it can make the back of my head feel like it is caving in."
—male, age 43

Gimme an O! Gimme Another O!

Just when you thought it was safe to roll over and go to sleep, know this: All orgasms were not created equal. Biology has provided boys with the capacity to stumble upon or even sleep through their first orgasms, and they keep a solid pace of routine orgasms through most of adulthood. Women usually have to work at having each orgasm on their own or with the help of a partner.

GETTING THE MOST BANG FROM YOUR BUCK

To maximize the orgasmic potential of a woman, guidance and communication are necessary, regardless of the level of enthusiasm and determination on the part of her partner. In fact, being too eager and determined can actually set back the progress. Because of the complexity of the physical setup and emotional components involved for women, satisfying orgasms with a partner are almost always a co-creation.

Female orgasms come from a variety of places, and perhaps most importantly, the mind. Most women agree that the connection with her partner is what most enhances her sexual experience. Strong attraction combined with mutual trust and respect lead to the openness that can make orgasms exceptional and elicit a variety of reactions including multiple orgasms, vivid mental images, out-of-body experiences, and female ejaculation.

CAMP CLITORIS

When men ask us the best way to get their lassies back to the game of sex, our advice is to ask for guidance from their partner and keep the clitoris on the radar even during intercourse. With over 30 years of sexual coaching under her belt, Betty Dodson concludes, "There remains no question in my mind that the clitoris, with its eight-thousand-plus nerve endings, remains a woman's primary sexual pleasure organ."

Dr. Susan Bennett describes why the clitoris plays such a starring role in orgasms. "The vagina is not the female version of the penis. The clitoris is the equivalent of the penis, and is, in fact, the same size as the penis. It's a complex, large structure five inches in length that is mostly hidden in the pelvis. From the tip of the clitoris, legs extend deep into the pelvis, where they attach to each side of the pelvic wall. The bulbs of the clitoris are two columns of erectile tissue that surround the outer two-thirds of the urethra, which sits just anterior to the vagina. It is not just the tip of the clitoris that is sensitive. The most sensitive areas are two areas on top of clitoris: in a fan above it and right on top. The next most sensitive area is on the side, then below, then at the entrance to the vagina and lastly around the outer third of the vagina and the cervix. Additionally, the areas of sensitivity are different at different levels of arousal. Stimulation of this structure is obviously trickier than stimulation of the penis. The labius minora is the hood of the clitoris. Theoretically the friction of thrusting rhythmically tugs down on the hood and stimulates the clitoris to the point of orgasm. But in reality fewer than 25 percent of women have orgasms with intercourse and without other stimulation."

> *"People don't get it about the clitoris. It needs extra stimulation. Otherwise it's like inviting the most important person to your party and then nobody talks to her."*
> —female, age 51

> *"In addition to clitoral stimulation, I like simultaneous vaginal penetration. I know that there are many women who just need clitoral stimulation to get off and could be perfectly happy to not have anything in their vaginas, but that is not me."* —female, age 42

O, O, O YOUR BOAT

There is no way around it—orgasms transport. Some women report feeling like they are floating or flying elsewhere, transported back in time or even astral traveling to another planet altogether. Others describe a meditative feeling of being at one with their partner or with the universe. One woman describes a particularly powerful orgasm as giving her a feeling of being all done up in a 1920s ball gown walking down a staircase surrounded by browns, blues, and greens. Colors are a commonly reported feature in these uber-orgasms. Much of the time, the best stuff comes on the second, third, or even fourth orgasm, leaving an undiscovered realm for the single-orgasm girl, or for others who may have the capacity but no energy to pursue it.

Not to get greedy, and certainly one orgasm is light years better than none, but you may find it motivating to know how much potential is out there. Achieving multiple or more intense orgasms is a function of many factors including openness, comfort, and proximity to your sexual peak. For women, that can mean you are well into middle age before discovering your pleasure potential. The journey for men and women toward these bonus levels of pleasure for her starts with a mutual desire to please and a willingness to communicate.

"Initially, my girlfriend was not forthcoming about what she liked, but once she was having orgasms she was more able to relax, talk about it, and articulate what she liked. It was a matter of being patient, doing it, having enough time, and eliminating distractions and stress. Her appetite for orgasms increases the more she has them. Generally, it is about 15 minutes of foreplay for her and 15 seconds for me to get us to an equal place before having intercourse. We communicate in terms of percentages. Often, we are in positions that provide maximum stimulation for her and minimal for me until she is at 95 percent, then we get into a more comfortable position for both of us to have orgasms. Sometimes we have sex without intercourse. Sometimes she doesn't have orgasms. We mix it up over the course of the week, so by the end it is balanced. Giving orgasms adds to the general experience for me. It feels best when she is exhausted afterward and it is something we did together. I feel like The Man." —male, age 23

WHAT DO WE KNOW

Cindy: "In the last few years, I have had more powerful orgasms. Occasionally, I see flashes of blue-glass, geometric-shaped castles. Sometimes I see a series of distinct, modern art paintings flash quickly in my mind's eye during one single orgasm. I have no interest or background in modern art. I wonder if orgasms tap into parts of the brain that are not in full use."

Edie: "I don't trust that I could have multiple orgasms regularly so I don't invest in that regularly. I get the message that I should want more, and I feel like there is a lot of pressure to say you want more and try to have more, but for day-to-day sustainable sex I am honestly happy to call it good with one."

ADVANCED DEGREES

If you ask around the medical community, some doctors will tell you there is no such thing as female ejaculation or that the research is inconclusive. Considering that there are limited studies on female sexual function, it is not surprising that available scientific information about the phenomenon is limited and conflicting. "There is zero scientific funding for studies on women's sexuality, unless it is on sexual dysfunction," says Rebecca Chalker in *The Clitoral Truth*. However, ample reports from women who have experienced female ejaculation combined with anecdotal data from workshops for discovering orgasmic potential present compelling and consistent insights on the topic. There is disparity between the medical world and the reports from the trenches in the cause, source, and content of squirting. Recent studies indicate that female ejaculation is associated with the G-spot (see Orgasm Mechanics) and approximately 30 paraurethral glands. It is believed that female ejaculate or "squirt" is produced by the Skene's gland. "The Skene's glands are embedded in the paraurethral sponge. Among the 30 paraurethral glands, Skene's glands are the two that adjoin the anterior wall of the vagina."*

Technically the substance that sometimes shoots out of women during orgasm is not "ejaculate" in the male sense of the word. Some medical professionals insist the fluid is simply urine finding its way out at an inopportune time, while others conclude that it is lymphatic fluid of the vagina.

According to Betty Dodson, "As for the mysterious fluid, evaluations so far have focused on proving that it is not urine. The most recent research has found PSA (prostate specific antigen) in female ejaculate, a substance that does not appear in either male or female urine. For those women who thought they were peeing when they climaxed, the acknowledgment of squirting has vindicated them. But with all the publicity surrounding squirting too many women felt pressured to find this magic spot in order to improve their orgasms or to please their partners."

Possibly medical professionals are reluctant to acknowledge squirting as normal because it could create an expectation for women, giving one more extreme to which they might aspire. Adding to the feelings of sexual

---

* "Female Ejaculation: Fact or Fiction," *Current Sexual Health Reports*,
  Sandra R. Leiblum, PhD and Rachel Needle, MS. 2006

inadequacy for women is something we all aim to avoid. Niches of the porn industry that make a spectacle of women who can squirt on demand, and with enough distance to shame any guy impressed by such things, portray squirting as the Holy Grail of orgasms. One woman who has never experienced squirting admitted to feeling under-experienced when women at a workshop piped up with stories of drenching the bedcovers with sacred amrita juice. "I had a wee moment of feeling I'd been missing something in that department." Squirting is associated with multiple orgasms and the G-spot, but as more of an accompaniment than an enhancement to the sensation.

"My very first orgasm, alone, resulted in a flood of liquid, but that never happened again until my later 30s. The next two times there was a gush of liquid because I had actually peed the bed along with the ejaculation. Once I learned to make sure my bladder was empty before I had sex, I found that there is a distinct difference between urine and the squirting liquid. Squirting only occurs when I have the stamina to have three or four orgasms. It doesn't make the orgasms more intense (and changing the sheets is a hassle), but it does occur when I am in my highest state of arousal during or between multiple orgasms." —female, age 41

"Just a finger in the bum to tickle my prostate, and all hell breaks loose."
—male, age 42

BEYOND VESUVIUS

With so much focus on the quest for the female orgasm, levels of male orgasm get little attention. But the male orgasm also has its finer points, depending, among other things, on how aroused the man is and whether he lets buildup happen toward the point of no return or wants to orgasm right away. One 43-year-old man describes his different levels as being: "short and sweet—feels good but rushed; longer and harder—the feeling runs more throughout my whole body; really out of this world—takes a long time to orgasm and, upon orgasm, my balls feel as if they are banging against each other, my penis feels like it is part of my wife, and the orgasm feeling goes all the way from my toes through all my chakras and out the top of my head." Too bad they can't pack that in a little blue pill.

As mentioned in previous chapters, the way a woman responds can greatly affect the male experience. Case in point:

"When a girl gets really into it by talking, moaning, squirming, and putting effort in, it can really help enhance an orgasm. Putting me over the top is anything that can personalize or set me apart

in her eyes or that plays to my individual vanities. One highlight sexual experience was when she took off my pants and exclaimed, 'Damn, that is hot. Your cock is hot.' That felt great and definitely got me more worked up. Doggy style is definitely one of my favorite positions (must be something primal in men), and she went right to it. I had to start out thrusting slowly so I wouldn't come immediately. To compensate for my slow pace, I reached around and used my finger to massage her clitoris. She also made it a point to tell me how good it felt, when she was coming, and that she had never come that fast before. Needless to say, I am looking forward to having sex with her again." —male, age 23

ILLUSIONS OF GRANDEUR

One would think that male ejaculation is pretty standard, but porn flicks mess with our idea of what is normal. Like spurting blood in horror movies, the clever special effects team enhances male ejaculation, when in reality 75 percent of men ooze their ejaculation rather than launch. And unless they are fueled by the power of DSB (Deadly Sperm Buildup), the launchers generally don't go that far.

Porn fuels the notion that women are or should be turned on by the "cum shot." However, unlike seventh-grade pals under the bleachers, most women are not impressed by how far a man can shoot his ammo. In fact, the prospect of it becoming a housekeeping issue—flying semen hitting the curtains, drenching the pillowcase, or landing in our hair—is probably more of a setback than a turn-on. There are certain aspects of porn that we find less than instructive in the big picture of healthy sex lives—we think the "money shot" is one of them.

WET DREAMS

Just as the levels of male orgasms are not often acknowledged, female wet dreams don't get much press. Although less common than in males, plenty of women describe enviable experiences that involve sexy dancing, long-lost heart-throbs, or even people to whom they are not attracted to in real life. These dreams are not necessarily gushy and wet, but often throbbing and splendid.

"I am the queen of wet dreams. If I sleep naked I am bound to have one. I call it a freebie. Such a bonus, no boner involved and no sleep lost." —female, age 34

ANAL SEX

And now, our vanilla disclaimer. We're not the ones to give you your back-stage pass. However, websites, videos, TV shows, books, and/or magazines aplenty will show you the way. We have heard from a few of those who are righteous about having a butt plug or anal beads during intercourse and a good number of women say they like anal sex. One study states that 35 percent of people have tried anal sex at least once and given the high number of nerve endings in the anus, this is undoubtedly a highly erogenous zone for some people. This is a broad topic with many strong opinions on both sides, but our comparatively modest mission is to encourage couples to start enjoying sex again or more often. The doorbell happens to be at the main entrance, and we are not equipped to accommodate the entire floor plan.

BOTTOM LINE

Orgasms can be good, great, or mind-blowing. They can stand alone or as a chain of events. There are some great pleasure zones all over the body, and once you and your partner are comfortable with the basics explore them at your leisure.

WHY YOU SHOULD CARE

Orgasms take the edge off everything. In the words of one 37-year-old woman who admits that pesky marital issues can feel oppressively complex: "A good fuck takes care of a lot of stuff that needs to be cleared up."

WHAT YOU CAN DO

Practice, practice, practice. The complete book of orgasms will never be written so get started on your own research, but don't let a complicated flight plan detour your mission. The clitoris is the ultimate source of pleasure for women. Be open to all areas of stimulation and you may find some interesting unexplored terrain. Whether you choose to pursue PhD-level research in orgasms by ferreting out uncharted erogenous zones, or stick with the tried-and-true clitoral orgasms, prepare yourself to evolve over time. Women who are "lined up" for orgasms during intercourse sometimes have issues down the road when their partner's performance changes, so keep an open mind to the need for a broad-ranging study to stay current in your orgasm curriculum. Figure out what works for you, run with it until it doesn't work anymore, and then dive into your next degree.

♀ ♂

"I faked orgasms with old boyfriends because the sex was like a bad amusement park ride. It's not going to get better the more times you go 'round—so throw your arms in the air, scream (even if you are ready to hurl), and get off as soon as it comes to a stop." —female, age 36

"Why would a woman want to reinforce something that I am doing that isn't working?" —male, age 26

Faking It: The Inhumane Option

Faking orgasms is a seemingly harmless quick fix for what can compound into a long-term crisis of trust. Many women have done it, do it, or wished they could do it, either as a way to end an unpleasant or unsatisfying experience, to make their men feel like champs, or simply to get that much closer to coveted sleep. Any man who has seen *When Harry Met Sally* knows how convincingly a woman can fake an orgasm. Whether or not you admit it to yourselves, you men have most likely been had on that score a time or two. The practice of faking is equal parts delusion and dishonesty.

Indeed part of the ease with which women can fake comes from the fact that men are so heavily invested in their ability to satisfy women that it is relatively easy to offer up a believable act. The question is not why men believe it—who can blame them for wanting to believe, not only in their prowess, but also in their partner's pleasure? The more vexing question is why women use faking to take advantage of men's desire to please.

WHY WOMEN FAKE

"Many women who never achieve orgasm through intercourse believe there is something wrong with them, that they are 'frigid,' even if they are capable of reaching orgasm through oral or tactile stimulation. Their partners may feel inadequate and frustrated that they cannot bring their women to orgasm. This is possibly why so many women fake orgasms at some point in their lives." —Dr. Susan Bennett

Faking can come from a wonderful loving place, from a woman's sincere desire to make her man feel vital, and to reciprocate his concern for her pleasure with an appropriate level of satisfaction. That's still no excuse. As much as it feels like a harmless white lie in the moment, it is a cop-out—a way to avoid explaining why you aren't getting around the bend, or asking for help in getting there. This can be an especially common solution among women who don't know or are unwilling to explore what works for them. One woman who thinks faking is "silly" sees it as more of a downward-spiraling communication problem between two people who sincerely want to please each other. By avoiding the truth they get less in touch with each other's needs and perpetuate the problem.

> *"I am always concerned about pleasing the woman I am with, and I hope that she does not have to fake orgasms, but I am not naive enough to believe that I can help her achieve an orgasm every time we make love."*
> —male, age 42

Another 23-year-old woman who gets turned on by her partner's confidence justifies faking as a way to keep him from feeling insecure and self-conscious: "I get enough orgasms. Getting off isn't a problem in our relationship. It doesn't hurt anyone if he thinks he is the man."

For those who can't get no satisfaction, faking perpetuates the problem.

> *"While 44 percent of men say their female partners always have orgasms when they have sex, 22 percent of women say they always have orgasms when they have sex."* —Marshall Miller and Dorian Solot, authors of *I Heart Female Orgasms*

> *"I never wanted to challenge my previous boyfriend's manhood, so I let him believe that he was great and I was satisfied. I remember feeling left out of the club, feeling that something was wrong with me. Eventually, I fessed up and then he began to feed me books on female orgasm, masturbation, etc. I learned that I was normal."* —female, age 36

AND WHY MEN FAKE

Though they are up against a much tougher task given the telltale bodily fluids involved, men have been known to fake orgasms as well. To be sure, these reports come mostly from young bucks in situations where alcohol or other psychotropic substances facilitate the illusion. Their motives—of reaching resolution and rewarding their partners' efforts or not hurting their feelings—are usually the same.

"For me, shower sex isn't that great, even though I push for it every time I get in the shower with someone. Blow jobs in the shower might as well not exist. She could go Scuba Steve for an hour with no results. I have faked orgasms in the shower just so she feels like we have not spent 20 minutes in vain." —male, age 21

WHY NOT TO FAKE

Reinforcing his false confidence and sacrificing your own pleasure isn't helping either of you in the long run. If you are not with a life partner, you are literally screwing him for the rest of his life by not alerting him to the shortcomings of his technique. When he finds someone who doesn't fake, his delusion and the ensuing letdown is going to be even more damaging to his psyche. Faking, whether under the guise of kindness or laziness, is inhumane.

"When a female friend of mine told me she was faking orgasms most of the time with her boyfriend, I told her she was cruel. She was so deep in the relationship that if she admitted she was faking, she would have severely shamed him. They recently broke up, and she has unleashed him into the world thinking he has all the right moves, when in fact they are useless. Cruel."
—male, age 23

"I bust her on it when she fakes or lies about it. But I did it once when I had to get up early and she wanted to have sex. I rallied, and didn't even come, but I told her I did."
—male, age 22

"If someone I really care about fakes an orgasm, I am offended and embarrassed. I like doing a good job, and when a girl fakes it I feel as though I didn't do my part. In fact, it can be pretty emasculating. If it's a one-night stand it still feels shitty to have a girl fake it, but I do not care nearly as much. In the end, I don't ever want a girl to fake an orgasm. I haven't done my part and from a selfish standpoint, I might not be as good as I thought I was. It is a blow to the pride." —male, age 22

We are here to tell women that, even in bed, honesty is the best policy. Men are mostly hurt and annoyed by faking. One man explains that letting him do something that doesn't feel good and then pretending that it does is simply "bad training," and adds that there is no better way to get him to repeat a good skill than to have a real orgasm. Men feel worse about themselves if a woman fakes to make them feel good. One man describes how it leaves a hole in the experience if one is only pretending to be satisfied. They would much rather be part of a true orgasmic experience than the Hollywood version, but they need your guidance.

HUMANE ALTERNATIVES

Many men report that the most erotic feelings they have revolve around arousing a woman and providing orgasms. They say that when their partner has or starts to have an orgasm, it makes them climax sooner. Most women learn this about men pretty quickly, and it is one of the reasons many women of all ages report that they fake orgasms. Both sides can do their part to eliminate the faking scourge. When men get comfortable with the idea that they are helping *cause* rather than *give* orgasms their success rate goes up. "Achieving" is the perfect word for the female orgasm as it is the hard-won reward for a team effort. A man should be proud of himself for contributing to the crescendo rather than feel wholly responsible for giving it. The idea of co-creating orgasms—rather than giving or receiving them—eases the tension by shifting the pressure from one to both partners.

The most direct remedy is to speak up and say what you need, that is of course after exploring and discovering what gets you aroused and over the top. Such communication makes you both better lovers by reinforcing the comfort level in your relationship.

> "Sometimes I say today's not my day (for an orgasm). It makes him more excited when I do have an orgasm, and I usually do, but I never fake them."
> —female, age 24

> "I have never faked an orgasm, so maybe that is why I am getting sleep."
> —female, age 43

> "My wife usually cannot orgasm during intercourse (it's a mechanics thing), but we always make sure she gets hers through other creative means." —male, age 44

> "What is the point of faking orgasms? Instead be confident and tell your partner what you like. I mean, if you feel comfortable enough to let a guy put his penis in your vagina, why should it be awkward to say, 'hey move your penis (or finger) a little to the left?'" —female, age 42

MOVING RIGHT ALONG

Sometimes a man is trying so hard to move things along that the orgasm process backslides. If you absolutely do not want to take the time to reach orgasm, say so or figure out ways to move it along for both of you. Men are often so fixated on slowing themselves down that they sometimes go overboard with fancy finger and tonguework making the moment last for women. Camping out on the pre-orgasmic side of Climax Ridge for a really long time is portrayed in literature and on film as especially erotic, with the wait enhancing the ultimate reward. In reality, teetering on the brink can be annoying to the point of being painful. The object for all is to get over the ridge to the other side of the mountain in a reasonable amount of time. There are all sorts of ways to accelerate the process if needed, but do not confuse speed with pressure and never underestimate the power of a light touch. Less direct clitoral contact—slightly to the side—can have the best results. Sometimes the slightest and lightest movement can send an orgasm right over the edge. The speed can be fast, but sometimes when there is too much pressure on the clitoris, the building orgasm can get snuffed.

"If a blow job is taking too long, I just pop a finger up his ass, and it's all over."
—female, age 27

"My husband tries to hold back to give me just one more orgasm even if I have had three or four. When my arches are cramping, hips ache, and I am exhausted, I speed things up by working the kegels and reaching around with my hand to cup his balls and put pressure on his perineum. That always sends him." —female, age 41

MAKING THE MOST OF THE NIPPLE EFFECT

The nipples help move things along for some women (and some men, actually), at different stages of life, or at different levels of arousal. The most current studies indicate that female arousal, once accessed, fosters continued sexual desire that allows previously unwelcome stimuli—to the breasts for example—to now be enjoyed. Reportedly 1 percent of women can have orgasms with nipple stimulation alone—for some women the nipples are like extensions of the clitoris. For others the nipples offer no extra stimulation ever, are overly sensitive, or only respond at certain times. Handling them too aggressively or too soon is counterproductive. The key is to find out where your partner is on this timing/touch continuum.

"Before babies, my nipples were part of the game but not huge factors. While nursing, I could barely stand having them touched. Once nursing was over for good, they became the kicker zone. He can't start with them but once aroused, nipple stimulation—from his mouth, hand, or even a rough elbow—can advance things, enhance things, and ultimately be the thing that sends me over the edge."
—female, age 41

BOTTOM LINE

Women who make it a policy not to fake, and men who encourage honesty regardless of their egos, are on track to a consistently more satisfying sex life. Is it ever okay to fake? Women, if you are getting pestered beyond belief, then he deserves it. Men, for all the faking that's been done by women, you deserve a few hall passes. For both, if you're trying out for a big role and your partner is the casting director, go nuts.

WHY YOU SHOULD CARE

We want to please each other, and feel good about our abilities to please each other. But faking—however rationalized or well intentioned—can erode a relationship like any other form of dishonesty.

WHAT YOU CAN DO

Men: Ask, ask, ask for guidance. Encourage her to be honest, ask for specific directions to figure out how to move her along toward orgasm, or give her an out. Remember what worked on a given day may not have the same effect on another day (see Drive Differential and Gimme an O!). Orgasms are great but so are a lot of other things about sex and intimacy. Sometimes it's just not meant to be, so try not to take it personally.

Women: Be honest and think beyond the moment. If you're just not getting there and don't care to make it happen, be polite but honest and say so. "That was nice," may not be what he wants to hear, but he will get over it. He will not get over discovering, years into your relationship, that he actually hasn't been satisfying you. Faking it means you're going to have to live the lie for a long time. The sooner you come to terms with it, the better for you both. Even with all hands (his or hers) on deck (the clitoris) during intercourse, many women are unable to have an orgasm without the stimulus of a vibrator. If your journey to paradise is too long to fit your lifestyle, get yourself teamed up with the perfect vibrator (See Taking Matters Into Your Own Hands).

WHAT DO *WE* KNOW?

Cindy: "I am way too greedy to fake orgasms. If I get to a certain level of arousal, there is no question that I am going all the way one way or another. If the timing isn't working, I am not afraid to assist."

Edie: "I don't know anything about faking. Back in the day it crossed my mind that it might be the polite thing to do, but ultimately I'm much too lazy to fake."

♀ / ♂

"Good sex is like good bridge. If you don't have a good partner you'd better have a good hand."
—Mae West

"Don't knock masturbation—it's sex with someone I love."
—Woody Allen

Taking Matters Into Your Own Hands

While we were interviewing a college kid about masturbation, he was visibly embarrassed, not only to be talking to two middle-aged women about it, but also to be admitting his need for it. He carefully explained that due to a long-distance romance he had to resort to masturbation, and asserted his sincere belief that his days of jacking-off would be over as soon as he had a live-in girlfriend, or certainly by the time he was married. At that point in the interview, though we didn't have the heart to break it to him, we were struck with the same thought: "He thinks this is temporary." Our advice to any young buck on the topic of masturbation: Keep up the skills.

Self-stimulation is widely regarded as being primarily within the male domain and men readily admit to its practice. One college man describes it as more of a training mechanism: "Jacking-off is about maintenance and building stamina, otherwise you go off like a rocket." Another man recalls his sexually formative glory days in high school: "Sometimes I'd binge when I was avoiding homework and do it three or four times a day. The last bust required hard work with a tired hand, and my ass sweating."

MASTUR AND MISTRESS BATING

There is so much anecdotal evidence on the relative imbalance between male and female desire for sexual frequency that, even before our research confirmed it, we firmly believed that for men, "releasing the hostages" through masturbation is a virtual necessity to keeping the peace in the typical household. We also expected to find that women in long-term relationships aren't looking for more ways to get off. Splat! Another assumption bites the dust. In many cases, the emotionally and physically easiest way for women to reclaim sexual desire is with a little private practice. Here's the story from a 33-year-old mother of two.

"After I stopped working and was at home with two toddlers I became very depressed, and unsure of who I was in this new role of stay-at-home mom. I did not know what being a good mother meant, and felt like I was not making progress in any direction. I resented my husband for having his own business, creating his own happiness, and being able to be good and productive every day in very measurable ways—financial and otherwise. My feelings about not working and my new status (or perceived lack thereof) in life were impacting our family and certainly my sex life.

"I thought one way that I could work on getting back into the swing of having sex with my husband was to remind myself of how pleasurable sex can be. With some regularity on the two mornings a week that I dropped my boys to their pre-school programs, I would stop at a convenience store for a large coffee and get all jacked up on caffeine while I drove home.

"By the time I got there I was alert and eager for 'action.' I immediately headed up to our bedroom and began my morning of solitude by unplugging the fan by the bed, then plugging in my own adult toy. That began my sex "therapy" session. My immediate goal was achieving an orgasm, and ultimately, perhaps ironically, achieving a better sex life with my husband. Once I was finished with the task at hand, so to speak, I returned the toy to its top-secret location, re-made the bed, and carried on with my day.

"After a few rounds of this, I felt better enough to make an effort to enjoy being intimate with my husband. Occasionally, as he plugged in the fan before bed I noticed a puzzled look on his face, which reminded me that I needed to cover my tracks better. Inevitably I forgot to do this a few more times and finally one night my husband asked why the fan was always unplugged. Without missing a beat I blamed my then two-year-old: 'He's constantly getting into everything, taking stuff apart—that's what the days are like around here . . .' One night while my husband and I were out to dinner talking about funny sex stories I came clean with the fan/

plug issue, to clear my two-year-old's name. Now I am clearer with my husband about things like self-image that can thwart good sex. We are in a good way and hopefully will continue to be. It's a work in progress—one day at a time."

GEARING UP FOR THE ORIGINAL SAFE SEX

Most of us are brought up believing that masturbation is such a cardinal no-no that it carries a huge sense of guilt. If you can get over that, however, self-love is the safest affair you can have and can be darned good therapy. Certainly the practice is a standard mental health measure for singles. But masturbation also has its place later in life, getting you through droughts caused by illness, travel, fatigue, annoyance, or whatever other barriers to sex inevitably crop up between couples. One group of male and female friends—all of whom had been with their respective partners for over 10 years—determined they had each had more orgasms from masturbation than from sex during their relationships. And they say kids take up all their free time.

For men, it's hard to improve on the price and convenience of the original masturbation gear—the hand. For women the hand is equally convenient and men rarely object to its introduction.

"If it's not happening, I throw my hand in the mix, and always have one. My women friends complain that they don't have orgasms, and I tell them to masturbate at the same time. I think some are too shy about it. With all the pressure to have sex, it would put me over the edge if I didn't have an orgasm." —female, age 43

For effortless amusement the tool of the trade is the vibrator, the multifaceted sex toy/therapist. Many women use them as a way to acquaint or reacquaint themselves with their bodies. "The first time I have sex, I meet you with my vibrator," says a 44-year-old divorced woman. "If you can't handle that, you can't have sex with me." To the men who seem threatened or perhaps shell-shocked at this statement, she continues: "This is what works for me now. If that changes you will be the first to know but for now I can't have an orgasm without a vibrator. That's just the way it is."

To the uninitiated, a cyber trip to Eve's Garden (www.evesgarden.com) or Good Vibrations (www.goodvibes.com)—one-stop shops for all your sex tool needs—will enlighten you to the variety of options available. Top sellers like the Hitachi Magic Wand can even be explained away to curious children and unexpected visitors as a massager. The two-speed Wand—known as the "Cadillac of Vibrators"—has two settings: low and overwhelming. You could sand a deck with this rig. And its size can be down-right scary unless you understand that the shaft is not meant to penetrate you. As one devotee notes, "It probably doesn't need to be as big as a wine bottle but it is . . . and it works through ANYTHING (some shops have a separate side room where you can try it out, over your clothes). I also tried the Pearl and the Rabbit. Lame. Mr. Happy (the Magic Wand) is the only one for me." To each her own, and we really mean it—do not share these.

Naming your vibrator seems to be a necessary step to sealing your relationship to it. One woman goes nowhere without "Pinky Tuscadero," in her satchel. It's important to note that vibrators may be the provenance of their "master's domain," but, used appropriately, they can also bring couples closer, not only by increasing a woman's sexual awareness but also by becoming a shared asset, much like a favorite pet.

While this may not conjure up your ideal image of intimacy, many couples have made it clear to us that packing heat has some serious advantages. Furthermore, as an enhancement it doesn't detract from the basic pleasure of sex.

> *"Men should know that a vibrator is maintenance, not a surrogate.*
> *Sex with a vibrator is a zillion times better than just using the*
> *vibrator to get an orgasm. I'm very tactile. I like all the sensations.*
> *The best sensations are my arms on his back, the sort of cuddle plus,*
> *and the entwining. Without that it's not exciting. I want my hips*
> *to be heaving and hot-sweat physicality. That's where the vibrator*
> *comes in. It allows you to be physical and sexual." —female, age 46*

Sold! With a case of Astroglide. Some couples credit vibrators with reinvigorating their sex lives, like the ultra-conservative 50-year-old woman who found her relationship stuck in the mud because of her disappearing sex drive. Her friends dragged her to her first porn shop and showed her exactly what to get. Now her husband insists she take it everywhere. He even let her pack it in his suitcase when they headed separate ways after a vacation, leaving him with some tense moments going through Customs.

For many women, vibrators provide the first awareness to the pleasures of sex. "It was a formative thing for me to realize that I don't have to wait around for an orgasm during sex. I don't think you should have to grin and bear it or think there is something wrong with you."

TAKING CHARGE

Generally, men get turned on by seeing women—alone or with company (even better)—touch themselves. And though men may fantasize that women are similarly aroused by such performances, we have to tell you that not many women report being turned on by watching their man masturbate. Most women are really okay with the reality that male masturbation has to happen, but don't bank on them wanting a front row seat.

That lack of voyeuristic interest does not mean lack of interest in experiencing her own pleasure. Interest in female self-stimulation is evidenced by the popularity of masturbation workshops like the one run by sex educator Betty Dodson, author of *Sex for One: The Joy of Selfloving* and *Orgasms for Two: The Joy of Partnersex*. Dodson delves right into the idea that women need to own their orgasms to have reliably good sex. Said one workshop participant: "It was the most informative thing I'd ever done. I brought a friend who was visiting me in New York City from Europe. She was a little surprised at what I'd planned for our weekend but it was great. There were adult women in every decade, including a 70-year-old woman who had her first orgasm recently. Her husband had died and a man in her retirement community wanted to give her oral sex. She felt 'something fluttering down there' and wanted to learn more."

> *"I have a friend who gave me masturbation advice in the car. She stopped and drew a full diagram of the vagina. It was a huge help."*
> —female, age 24

Fortunately, learning more about the art of masturbation does not require matriculation to a workshop. If you're lucky, it can only take a little helpful advice from your friends:

> *"My brother caught me early on and gave me feedback on my technique. He said I should use my whole hand rather than just my two fingers and thumb. I was so embarrassed, but he was right."*
> —male, age 27

Masturbation is not only about whiling away the long summer days on a hammock but about learning how your body works and responds. With enough practice, you can chart out your own detailed flight plan and, like this woman, pass those coordinates along with NASA-like precision: "Being on top with my boobs in the air like in 'those movies' doesn't work for me. I've never had an orgasm on top. For me, a 35-degree entry point is Nirvana."

THE GUILT FACTOR

Feelings of confidence and empowerment that accompany successful self-stimulation are increasingly common among women, but they don't ever

> *"The adage that if you masturbate before you have sex later in the day, it will help you not come too fast is somewhat true, but the feeling is not the same. I feel guilty playing with myself so ensuing sex is not as satisfying for me even though I stay hard longer the second time."*
> —male, age 43

quite erase the underlying sense of guilt we have about masturbation. Even men, despite the broader cultural acceptance of masturbation as normal behavior, cling to the guilt.

One 38-year-old male explained that he had to stop masturbating cold turkey because he had "all kinds of bad luck" every time he masturbated. When pressed about the types of consequences he admitted to "speeding tickets." Certainly pulling over first is a good idea. The same goes for the woman who resorted to masturbating on a long road trip to stay awake. "Every time I looked at the speedometer I was going about 45 miles per hour." And it goes without saying on interstate travel—beware of big rigs and their elevated drivers.

If you're still looking to absolve yourself of the guilt associated with masturbation, the medical community condones the practice, and often even flat-out encourages it. Says one gynecologist: "It may not be a good counseling method but sometimes I have to tell people that, when a partner is unhealthy or has had surgery, it is perfectly reasonable to have sex on your own." The same doctor admits that the practice can be pathological, as it was for the guy who showed up in the ER with a chafed penis from too much self-love, or the college basketball player who couldn't make it on the court because he couldn't stop masturbating.

LETTING IT ALL HANG OUT

According to Dr. Hilda Hucherson, gynecologist and author of *What Our Mothers Never Told Us About Sex*, the number-one reason why women don't enjoy sex is because they don't know their bodies. She recommends "strutting" proudly and sexily around the house naked, and then setting time aside each day to "rediscover yourself" by massaging your body and finding your erogenous zones. This meshes pretty well with our theory that you have to know how to please yourself to be able to teach your partner how to please you. Says Hucherson: "It's important that you do it yourself and not depend on someone else to give it to you. It's in you, your sexual energy, not with him."

Strutting and stroking and vibrating is all well and good, but a word to the wise if you are in the market for tools of the trade: Go to the right store because all appliances are not created equal. The best gear made with the safest materials can be found in female-owned and female-operated sex shops such as a-womans-touch.com, evesgarden.com, goodvibes.com, babeland.com, and goodforher.com, among others.

BOTTOM LINE

If you've got the itch there's no harm scratching it. Exploring and knowing your own terrain won't hurt your sex life and will most likely improve it. Try it—nobody's looking.

WHAT DO WE KNOW?

Cindy: "After I found the doorbell, I masturbated every night for a year. Now that I am spinning three careers and three kids, it's hard to make time for it, especially since my husband is ready and willing. It takes effort to keep sex on the priority list, therefore I save my orgasms for game days."

> *"I had a boyfriend once who was into sex toys. I had a vibrator at that time and I was constantly worried that I would get killed in a car accident and die and my mother would go through my stuff and find the vibrator. In the midst of mourning me, my mother would be thinking that I was some sort of sex freak!"*
> —female, age 43

Edie: "The downside of being the girl that guys wanted to marry but not date was obvious. The upside was that I got to know myself *very* well. As someone who endured more single stretches than the average female, I can't see the anything wrong with masturbation. Why not? It's free, it's easy, it's clean, and nobody gets hurt."

♀ / ♂

"I don't like the idea of oral sex, but it sure feels good when I'm getting it."
—female, age 37

"Back in high school, when my girlfriend would only give me a blow job, all I wanted was to get laid. Now that I am married and can get laid regularly, all I want is a blow job." —male, age 42

Oral Sex: Put Your Honey Where Your Mouth Is

There is a reality-checking cartoon that circulates among married couples sometime after their proverbial honeymoon is over. In it we read the thought bubbles over a smiling couple at the altar. The man's bubble reads, "Free blow jobs for the rest of my life!" The woman's bubble reads, "No more blow jobs for the rest of my life!" It sums up the prevailing stereotype that men fantasize about oral sex while women dread it or boycott it entirely. The reality lies somewhere in between.

AFTER "I DO" SOME DON'T

Certainly, plenty of couples do leave oral sex at the altar, but others keep it going strong. Some shift to using it more as foreplay than as the main event while others use it as a reward system. For others it is a way to give the man satisfaction around that time of the month or to give the woman satisfaction when the man has erectile issues. In both giving and getting some women delight in it, some endure it, and some want no part of it. Some people find it more intimate than intercourse, others find it less, and when it comes to swallowing, the jury is most definitely split. Almost all men say they like it when she swallows, while many women feel like it's a gag order.

In the post-Lewinsky era, oral sex is certainly much more openly discussed, though personal experiences are not exactly cocktail conversation.

At its best, oral sex is transporting for both partners, an erotic zing that offers a shortcut to the female orgasm, a pathway for multiple orgasms, and a way to achieve simultaneous orgasms. At its worst, oral sex is riddled with so much guilt, resentment, or unspoken desire that scores of men would rather risk their careers for it than nego-tiate for it at home. Bitterness oozes from men who feel that they are not getting enough of it and from women who feel goaded into perform-ing a "service." Guilt plagues men who feel they need to beg for it, and women who are unable to meet those needs enthusiastically.

> *"Blow jobs?! Weren't we done with that in college?"*
> —female, age 38

ONE-SIDED WONDER

It's messy business to separate this soup of issues into its ingredients, but it may well start with the basic fact that oral sex—except for the ergonomi-cally challenging "69" position—is an inherently one-sided act. One 22-year-old PBG male makes it abundantly clear that the best part about a blow job is the psychological aspect. "It's a dominant position for the guy, and it feels great. There isn't much more we can ask for," he explains, add-ing unabashedly, "and it's even better when she looks up at me. I don't know why."

Indeed, one-sided adoration seems too good to be true, until you real-ize that it is. Long-term relationships develop a sort of goodwill account that fluctuates with deposits and withdrawals by each partner. Couples who have an imbalance in their desire or willingness for oral sex often run into trouble managing their sex account. You will read a complete discus-sion of the sex account in Positive Balance in the next section, but for now it's important to understand that the one-sided aspect of the act of oral sex makes it especially vulnerable to the tit-for-tat syndrome. One woman's earliest sex advice from her mother was, "If you're giving it to him, he best be giving it to you!" However, the man who says, "Reciprocity has always been my mode of operating. You give, you get," needs to keep in mind that receiving oral sex is not necessarily a reward. Many women, though not op-posed to giving it, are simply not comfortable on the receiving end and feel ungrateful or embarrassed saying so—much less critiquing their partner's technique. Some say they only like to receive oral sex when they are feeling especially confident and comfortable with themselves and their partners.

"I truly don't mind—and even enjoy—giving oral sex to my husband because I know he likes it so much. As far as receiving goes, I've always

been a little self-conscious, so even when my husband is willing to do it I sometimes don't let him go there. I've never had an orgasm with oral sex because I'm too busy worrying what he's thinking." —female, age 34

"After childbirth, my wife was almost ashamed of the state of affairs, and didn't want me to have the visual. It was difficult for her to be aroused due to her own insecurity. And that definitely reduced the buzz." —male, age 42

APPRECIATION

Whether 'tis better to give or receive varies with each individual. Ideally, couples find a combination that is comfortable and satisfying for them both. Men and women agree that oral sex is most pleasurable when it is appreciated. The response of the partner is the arousing part, not necessarily the participation in the act in itself. One man explains that he is not as turned on by blow jobs anymore because they don't work for his partner: "I'd rather do something that fires her up." Another feels that the giving and receiving of oral sex requires enthusiastic participation to maximize the value delivered. "It is not fun to get a blow job if the performer's heart isn't in her work. Of course, that is also true of regular sex," he says.

> *"That is where you earn your jewelry—quick and easy."* —female, age 44

> *"When my friends' husbands do something really cool I tell them, 'he deserves a blow job for that!'"* —female, age 45

"When I was young I thought that the 'boxed lunch at the Y' was disgusting. Of course, I thought that sex was all about me back then. I have learned slowly but surely that, as in most areas of life, sex is better when you give and give freely, and without inhibition. Somewhere around age 30 I really started to enjoy the oral act, and now I must say that it is one of my greatest turn-ons. I have made a 180-degree turnaround because getting my partner heated up and excited is the biggest turn-on for me that I know." —male, age 44

FREQUENCY

On the topic of frequency, a general lack of communication leads us deep into the realm of assumptions. Men assume all their friends are getting more oral sex than they are getting, while women think their friends are giving more than they are giving. Both men and women often feel inadequate for not giving it more, while women (and even some men) feel abnormal for not wanting to receive it.

Many couples resort to policies to set their oral sex agenda. One woman admits she gives her husband a blow job once a year on his birthday, and sometimes skips a year because she, a) hates it; and b) thinks she is bad at it (which is a likely consequence of a). Another man has successfully negotiated his age equivalent in blow jobs over the course of the year as an annual birthday present. "It sort of makes me want to live until I'm 365." Another man,

> *"The biggest boost for me was to hear her say, 'Where did you learn that?!' My apparently wrong answer was, 'Lots of practice.'"*
> —male, age 42

whose wife had an "only on holidays" policy got himself an aggressive Hallmark calendar and all of a sudden they were celebrating Flag Day, Arbor Day, and Groundhog Day, among many others.

ORAL VS INTER

> *"Intercourse is like a two-person rowing scull, with both rowers working as a team to stay in rhythm and reach the finish line together. Oral sex is like a rowboat ride. One person does all the work and the other gets to kick back, hold the umbrella, and enjoy the view."* —male, age 38

Whether or not oral sex is better than intercourse generally depends on the delivery, the available alternatives, and the level of intimacy and arousal. Given the choice between one or the other, some men say blow jobs are a nice accessory but not the real thing.

One man admits he is lukewarm about giving oral sex at the beginning of a sexual encounter, but as his state of arousal rises his desire increases dramatically. For some women, giving oral sex feels so much more intimate than intercourse that it takes being more aroused to go there. Many men are offended at the lack of intimacy they perceive when they are being "bought off" with a blow job.

> *"Let's face it. If I were a dog, I would lick myself constantly."*
> —male, age 44

> *"I want to please her every time we have sex. When she doesn't want to take the time to have an orgasm, she gives me the preemptive blow job. It's nice, but she's blowing me off. I'd even prefer a fake."* —male, age 44

THE NAUGHTY APPEAL

Oral sex is undoubtedly a deterrent for men and women who grew up associating it with being dirty and shameful. For others the taboo aspect only strengthens its allure.

"Oral sex is outstanding. Its tainted image gives it appeal. You look down, the head is bobbing, you're thinking, 'I should be in a movie right now.' When offered oral sex, I am unable to politely decline. I always accept. Game on!!" —male, age 37

"It's a gift. I don't enjoy it as much as my husband does but its eroticism has its good points. It's something unexpected at an unexpected time—an enhancement when we're feeling a little extra frisky or kinky that reminds us of the early days of our relationship. A nice place to visit, but I don't have to live there." —female, age 40

HYGIENE

"Oral sex was the only way I could have an orgasm when I first had one at age 31. The 'odor' thing has always put a little edge of shyness on it for me." —female, age 71

Upkeep and hygiene play a major role in how people perceive the giving and receiving of oral sex, as well as the likeliness of making it a lovemaking staple. Some men are adamant in their preference of a "clean workspace" and interpret a fully or mostly waxed pubic zone as an invitation. Says one father in the trenches of bringing up young kids, "Waxing signals your husband that you are thinking about sex, that you are willing to groom the playing field to get it, and that you are just a little bit naughtier than you let on." Another less picky man reminds women never to underestimate the value of a shower and a trim: "It doesn't have to resemble a putting green, but it should also not look like a recently fertilized sod farm." Others attest that they have no problem blazing a path through the jungle. Men do swap stinky vagina stories, so as one man advises, "Any self-respecting, hopeful recipient of cunnilingus will proactively initiate and commit to a strong box-maintenance regimen." One previously scarred man urges women to "keep it clean and warn me if there are dangers (blood, infection, skank) down there."

For women it's a whole lot of effort to keep yet another area of our bodies tidied up for company. But if she is prepared, a woman is much more relaxed and able to enjoy it being part of the menu. Men, take note that

Fumunda ain't no picnic fare for women either. Both sides have their issues to deal with. The whole randy, camping, gamey, haven't-showered-in-three-days thing is so not sexy when you share the sheets.

"My husband used to come to bed with greasy hair, BO, bad breath, and nut scudge. With some persuasion he started showering, and I was all psyched for the clean guy. Somehow he always missed something key. When he remembered to floss, use soap under his arms, and clean the full genital area, he recognized a significant improvement in his sex life." —female, age 41

"My wife loves the combination of oat soap and Aveda aftershave I use on my face, so I used the same treatment on my crotch area. When she was giving me an oral 'warm up' to sex she noticed the luscious familiar smell, which I now call 'my concocktion.'"
—male, age 44

For some people, no amount of oat soap will whet the appetite for oral sex. They are simply not into it and women in this category are quick to point out that they don't call it a blow *job* for nothing. In any case a little forethought can go a long way. Men and women need to give each other fair warning, especially if you are working anything new into your routine.

A QUESTION OF TASTE

When introducing a new food to toddlers the experts say it takes 10 times before they acquire the taste for it, and at least another 10 before it gets into their repertoire. That may explain why some men who have a long history of giving oral sex are unfazed by the odor issue. Some men theorize that there is a point where the physicality of sex transcends into something more chemical, or even emotional. "Girls like their Daddy's BO, and guys like their wives' nether regions—how they smell, how they taste, the whole nine. . . . or at least they'd better if they want to get the party started," suggests one man. Another speculates that the palate matures—much like the unexplained transition from kids wanting ketchup on a hot dog to older people preferring mustard—easing the way for the enjoyment of giving oral sex.

"I think there is a primal center in the brain that can make associations that rework what is the perception of a sensory input based on goal-oriented behavior. In other words, if there is a treasure in the back of the cave, suddenly the bat turds smell good."
—male, age 43

"I have always very much enjoyed the smell. I am a primal, guttural creature hardly evolved beyond a rudimentary notochord. Eventually, even if you did not originally like the smell, it becomes associated with pleasure and you begin to be conditioned to like it more. This is all the more reason for men and women to have more sex."
—male, age 46

"Most women I know hate giving oral sex, and some love it. I have a friend who loves it. She told me to pretend it's a cherry popsicle. I had heard you were supposed to hold it in your hand and pretend it was the man you love and give it all the love you wanted to give him. My friend assured me, 'The cherry popsicle's better. Trust me, it works.' To me it's still the baloney pony." —female, age 41

GOING THE DISTANCE TO THE BIG O

Most people are first introduced to oral sex as a safer alternative to intercourse. Under those circumstances, going the distance is a reasonable expectation. However, as oral sex progresses from being a substitute for, to being a route to, mutual pleasure, and then on to being an accessory to intercourse, the rules tend to change. Most men report that they are willing, and in fact happy, to see their work through to full satisfaction. However, even when a couple has oral sex in their routine, many a woman feels the pressure of psychic waves from her partner urging her to "go the distance" and finish what she started. Some women relish giving that pleasure, down to the last drop, while others do not enjoy choking it down. Also, many women prefer transitioning to intercourse before blast off.

Finally, a note from your doctor: As we age and performance isn't what it used to be, oral sex may well move from being the sizzle to being the steak of your sex life. Dr. Susan Bennett says, "For some women who need deeper penetration for orgasm, oral sex gets in the way of concentration. But for most women oral sex is key. If your partner isn't good at cunnilingus, get a vibrator."

"We always start out with him giving me oral sex. I have my first orgasm and immediately we move to intercourse and both have orgasms. I am so used to our system that I feel cheated if I don't get at least two orgasms."
—female, age 37

BOTTOM LINE

Oral sex is an indulgent delicacy to some, repulsive to others. Even at its best, most long-term couples do not rely on it for

ORAL FEEDBACK: A BLOW JOB CRIB SHEET FOR WOMEN FROM THE PBG GUYS

- Use moisture. Wet lips and licking up and down the shaft is a great start.
- Lick the balls, which are very sensitive, at the start. Put one or both in you mouth or massage them with the other hand—this feels fantastic and makes our orgasm much more enjoyable.
- Put one hand on the shaft, and cup the balls and tickle behind them with the other.
- Coordinate hand and mouth. There is nothing worse than sucking up with the mouth and pulling down with the hand.
- No need for the death grip with the hand on the shaft unless we tell you to squeeze harder . . . you can suck pretty hard since the force there is much less.
- As much skin contact as possible.

BONUS, PORN STAR POINTS

- You don't have to swallow, but it is a nice touch.
- Most girls cannot deep throat, but those that can, should. Using just the mouth takes a long time and you have to be very good with that mouth.

A Special Note we can't resist: Those who *can* deep throat probably have had a lot of practice, and you might want to think twice about where you are sending your main man.

their sexual sustenance. It ranges from mind-blowing to tolerable to something you want to sweep beneath the rug. If you like oral sex and you're getting it, be happy. If you're not getting or giving it, you're not alone. Many couples thrive on it, while others have fully satisfying sex lives without it. It is all about finding a mutual comfort zone.

WHY YOU SHOULD CARE

Oral sex can function in a relationship along a full spectrum, from being a source of mutual pleasure to being a huge reservoir of guilt and resentment to being a non-issue. Exploring each partner's relative desire or lack of desire for it will optimize the role it plays in your sex life.

WHAT YOU CAN DO

No matter how carnal you feel, you're better off keeping oral sex respectful. It's

> *A guy should never put his hands on the back of her head while getting a blow job unless a lap full of puke turns him on.* —female, age 42

A FEW FAVORITE TECHNIQUES FOR PLEASING WOMEN

- Lick your ABCs: No-brainer way to cover the territory. The only draw-back to this technique is the tendency to hum along.
- Beware of the tongue. Some women prefer a flat tongue (think licking a frosty). The darting lizard tongue can be painful.
- The Nose Drag: The tongue is great but what can really take it over the top is dragging the bridge of the nose across the clitoris. Don't be surprised to hear, "What is that?!?" in a primal tone.
- Fingers: A couple of fingers working inside the vagina can enhance the pleasure.
- Double Play: Get her close to orgasm, then you can orgasm together, or better yet, give her a double, first by giving her oral sex then making the quick change-up pitch to intercourse.

Note: If it looks like the guidelines for women are less specific, it's because they are. Even if you don't ask for driving directions, ask for oral sex directions.

always good to be patient and grateful, and never appropriate to be pushy or greedy. Even for those who claim 'tis better to give than to receive, the pleasure for the giver is derived from the pleasure of the receiver. Keep that in mind when showing your appreciation. When trying to even up your sex account, know that oral sex can be fertile bonus territory, but don't assume your partner values the same currency. Do find out what really pleases him or her. For anyone who feels deprived or inadequate, take heart: it's never too late to learn. One woman heard about 69 from her sister as a 12-year-old and was repulsed by oral sex. She then took it up in her 50s and now, in her 70s, it is a key part of her lovemaking routine.

WHAT DO WE KNOW?

Cindy: "Before I started having sex, I was game for the full hummer. Now that we are short on time and sleep, I give a hummer to get things started, but then we move to intercourse. One of my guy friends said, 'Pierce. I don't buy the idea of women giving a hummer as a warmup to sex. A hummer is not called a hummer unless the deal gets closed.' My husband agrees whole-heartedly."

Edie: "The key thing about oral sex is preparation. If you aren't expecting it, it's sort of like your mother-in-law showing up unannounced when your house is a mess. It's tough to enjoy the visit when you're cringing about the disarray."

Section III:
Sex for the Long Haul
(In Search of Happily Ever After)

There are those who believe monogamy is an unnatural state, destined either to fail or leave us dissatisfied. We're taking that bull by the horns. Sex for the long haul is all about sustainability and a willingness to work together. Some things—like maintaining a certain appearance, sexual tension, or the ongoing delivery of affirmations—that you deemed critical for creating the fire become more trouble than they're worth. Meanwhile, things that are less apparent—such as how we communicate, show our respect, and share responsibility—reflect the core of our love, character, and connection, and make all the difference in how or whether we thrive, long term. Sex is only one part of the recipe for a successful, mutually satisfying long-term relationship, but it is a vital component that can either sweeten or sour the feast.

Denise Donnelly, associate professor of sociology at Georgia State University, has been studying involuntary celibacy for about 20 years. It all started when she watched an Oprah show on couples who were happy in sexless marriages. Immediately afterward she incredulously related the show to a close friend who, instead of agreeing with Donnelly on the improbability of such a scenario said, "I'd be happy if I never had sex again." Donnelly was so dumbfounded by the response and the concept that she decided to focus her PhD dissertation around one question: "Are there people who are happy in a sexless marriage?" Her answer, then and now (based on statistical evidence and her latest survey of 352 people in sexless relationships) is, "not many."

All manner of things can interfere with a couple's sex life: naturally differing sex drives, unresolved emotional issues, childbirth, aging, career stress, and just plain busy schedules. Getting off track and out of the rhythm of sex can even be seen as a natural stage of maturing and building a life together. Anticipating these phases and resolving to deal with them together is a key success factor for couples. Dr. Susan Bennett, through her lectures on Human Sexuality at Harvard, her gynecology practice at Massachusetts General Hospital, and 25 years of marriage, has had ample opportunity to observe and study the sexual aspect of long-term relationships:

"The problem with our generation is that we base our beliefs about our sexuality on male sexuality. The feminist movement said we are all the same. We wanted to be the same at work, the same as parents, the same physically and intellectually. The reality is that there are significant differences."

She notes that the pivotal work of Masters and Johnson created unrealistic expectations. Their model showed the path of male and female orgasm as being very similar, ideally resolving with simultaneous orgasm. The study, however, included only women who were self-selected as easily orgasmic and ignored the factor of desire. In reality, anywhere from 10 to 51 percent of women are affected by low desire. Consequently, our whole understanding of what is "normal" sexual response and desire is unrealistic, as are our expectations.

Men don't understand why their wives don't initiate sex, why mutually satisfying intercourse takes time, why their partners don't want to engage in eroticism. Women wonder where their libido is hiding, or they have ample drive but don't know how to get their needs met within the marriage. Neither men nor women can agree about where or if to put sex on the priority list, yet when ignored, sexual dissatisfaction commands a disproportionate amount of mental energy. Beneath much of the anxiety is a fear, compounded by poor communication, that married life is simply supposed to be boring as hell.

"Monogamy is a construct of society, but it sure is comfortable," says Bennett, who points out that in ancient societies men had multiple partners. She is nonetheless convinced that long-term relationships can work and that an active sex life is critical to success. "I lived the wild, hot, libidinous life with miniskirts and Jane Fonda boots. Then I had two kids late in life and nursed them for three years. I thought sex was a big pain in the butt. Then I got breast cancer at age 43 and lost my ovarian function. I know what it's like to have a profound disability on sexual function. I know what it's like to lose it. You can't ever take your partner or your sex life for granted."

Each partner in a couple needs to understand the other partner's needs—which are physiologically and emotionally unique, anticipate them, and meet them in a way that meshes with their lifestyle. We need to find ways to balance our give and take to assure each partner bears an equitable and acceptable load. And occasionally, we have to add a little spice to our recipe, by making the extra effort to plan an "away game"—a weekend escape, a faraway wedding, or an extended work trip to an exotic locale. Away games bring back the person we fell in love with and remind us that our need for intimacy extends beyond child making. Whether it's provocative emails during the day to him, surprising her with flowers, giving him two hours to go on a mountain bike ride, or folding the laundry unbidden by her to clear the decks for time together, there are little things we can do for each other every day to keep us pointed toward happily ever after.

♀ / ♂

"What I remember is the rough-and-tough, callused, all-business nipples from nursing. This was an issue for me because I have always felt lucky to be endowed with three clitorises, yet with the two northern headlights out, I had to depend on the south pole solely to bring on an orgasm. That was a lot of pressure for my clitoris—it was such a team player." —female, age 41

"I would describe getting back to sex after your wife gives birth like being a kid in the back of the car on a long trip: 'Are we there yet? Are we there yet?' Can we f^&% yet? With kids and careers and no sleep you just have to accept that sex requires planning." —male, age 39

Getting Back in the Saddle

Under any circumstances the road back to having a sex life after having a baby is tough. The OB's standard advice is to wait six weeks after giving birth to have sex. This is not a number created to drive men crazy. After six weeks is it safe to assume that the cervix has completely closed up and can maintain a sterile environment for the uterus. This also accommodates the average time it takes for the body to recover. First off, the uterus (which has morphed from a change purse to a large knapsack) and the vagina (which now resembles an udder) need time to recover and recede. It takes time for the bleeding to stop, the episiotomies and tears to heal, and the insides to resettle into their former digs. Add in cracked nipples, spurting breasts, a belly that feels like sponge cake, no sleep, and no time to shower, and you can glimpse the birth and post-birth factors that conspire against a woman's sex drive.

When there are extenuating medical situations for the baby or the mother, a sex life is not even on the radar at six weeks postpartum. Even if you are blessed with a fast recovery and a baby who sleeps a lot, it is still difficult to get back in the sex saddle. As one mother and nurse describes it vividly: "Too many people mistake six weeks as the jumping off point for returning to a 'normal' sex life. You now have a non-sleeping infant, milk everywhere, a house full of in-laws, and a hole in your ass the size of Texas. 'Normal' as anyone knows it is a thing of the past." Once you have physically healed, feeling mentally ready is a personal thing, complicated by rampant hormones and emotions, not to mention a perpetual borderline psycho state induced by sleep deprivation.

Giving birth is such a total turn-yourself-inside-out effort that a woman often wants to retract and retain any morsel of energy for herself. As a 54-year-old woman who still freshly recalls being postpartum exclaimed, "Erogenous zones? Forget it! Sex? Forget it! The thought of someone else needing my body put me over the edge. I had nothing left to give." Feeling like a beast of burden, constantly toting not only a helpless infant but also his twin-barreled, chest-mounted, life-support system, does not allow much room to take on anyone else's needs. A 50-year-old mother of grown children recalls, "After nursing, diapering, laundry, and figuring out motherhood all day, I finally find myself in bed cozy with a book and then one more person needs something from me? Give me a fucking break!!"

Beyond the physical exhaustion and pain, women have significant emotional hurdles to overcome before feeling any urge to share their bodies. One woman summed up the effect of her physical state on her mental state, "That first baby came out after three days of labor; I felt like I had a barn door between my legs—one that was sore, swollen, and a bit torn. How would that EVER again feel sexual, and how could I ever feel sexy?"

WHAT DO WE KNOW?

Cindy: "Our baby was 10 days old. I was perched on the edge of our bed trying to gather strength for the day ahead after nursing all night. Having drained the nursing jugs, the baby was sprawled out in a drunken slumber, but the breasts were still unmanageable. This was especially true during the transition into a nursing bra from the loose sleeping bra that merely acts as a hammock to keep the absorbent nursing pads in place as well as a safety net to keep the breasts from escaping down the side of the bed, snuffing out my baby, and rolling into the neighbor's yard. As I began the contortionist climb into the thick-strapped, quadruple-hooked nursing bra, and inserted fresh nursing pads under the Dumbo-like flaps that hooked below the shoulder, I caught sight of my pasty white triple-rolled belly hanging over a giant pair of granny panties specially acquired to hold my tremendous sani-

ADVICE FROM THE MIDWIFE

Sex can be likened to labor in that the main task for many women in our culture is to get their brain out of the way of their body, and surrender to the force of the experience. "I would say about 50 percent of women have some discomfort as they get back into the swing of things after they have a baby. My advice is that they should:

1) Use lots of artificial lubricant;
2) Continue with gentle intercourse;
3) Stop if it is painful and wait a week and try again. Very occasionally (and this is more likely with a significant amount of perineal stitches) a woman will need to do perineal massage—or rather have her partner do it—to desensitize.

Emotional issues are common in postpartum as well. It can be a bit scary to think about anything going in and out of there after birth. Obviously tension will inhibit sexual response, lubrication, etc. As the saying goes, the primary erogenous organ is the brain. I feel it's my responsibility to convince women that birth is a normal natural function, and that women's bodies are not only meant to do it, but meant to return to normal afterward. If one approaches sex as a chore, it will be a chore. If one approaches it as an opportunity for positive sensual exchange, hopefully it will be just that. Practice does not always make perfect, but no practice will definitely affect your game."

—Laurie Foster, CNM, CPM, MS

tary napkin in place. Peeking from beneath the belly was the jungle landscape of a wildly overgrown bikini zone and legs that had been unshaven for weeks. At that moment, Bruce walked in the door from the bathroom and stopped in his tracks, his eyes alight at the sight of my partially naked body. His was the face of pure desperation. Clearly his standards had shifted during the postpartum drought, which had only just begun."

Edie: "I was so focused on my panicked fear of labor that I was blindsided by all the postpartum issues of the childbirth process. Everything 'down there' felt like lead and the bleeding was out of a bad horror movie. For some dumb reason I decided to get on a bike after three weeks because I'd heard of a friend who bounced right back. Bad mistake. It hurt like hell and set me back. You *must* listen to your own body on this."

THE POSTPARTUM MALE

The emotional toll of birth is not reserved for women, though few people in the process acknowledge the tsunami of emotions that engulf men during the ordeal (miraculous event, yes, but an ordeal nonetheless). There is the feeling of helplessness throughout delivery, the attention focused first on mother then on child, as well as the somewhat horrific scenery on which the man is forbidden to comment. Here's what one new dad recalled:

"I had become rather well versed in the particulars of the 'gine in the weeks before as we were doing some 'stretching' exercises and vitamin E oil massage to prep for the big event. My wife would lie on her back, legs spread, and I would soften up the top of the taint with some oil, then use my thumbs to pull things this way and that. It was such a clinical chore that the region lost some of its stature as a sexual zone.

"During birth she tore in a major way—almost to the rectum and it became my job to monitor how everything was healing because she couldn't get a good view down there. When I looked at the stitches, swelling, discoloration, and hair all I could offer was some sort of 'making progress' comment.

"When the doctor did the routine Q&A about sex and birth control I could safely assure him that sex was not going to be an issue for a while. I still had a vivid image of the stiff, navy blue 'v' ends of the surgeon's knot on the sutures poking up above the puckered, bruised skin and into the pubes. Having that pop in the TV screen of the mind is all it takes to bring the libido to a screeching halt."

MAKING THE LEAP

A return to sex is at the back of the woman's mind, while the six-week countdown is the beacon of salvation for the man. He deserves it after all. He's been patient and kind and loving and he's the father of this miraculous baby. Of course, you love him even if it pisses you off that he is anticipating sex like a starving coyote. Persuasive as they sometimes seem when it comes to wanting sex, men say it is no fun to have sex with a woman who is doing him a favor. Men want the desire to be mutual. Furthermore, after the basic healing has occurred they are less discriminating about physical appearance than women in their foreign, postpartum bodies assume.

Even if you can't imagine wanting anything more than Pop Tarts, dry breast pads, water, and sleep, eventually the time comes to get back in the saddle. Sooner or later you have to take that leap. The key at this point is to try to recall the pleasures of sex. Once you can recall even one pleasurable encounter, there is hope of returning to that feeling of connection. This is a dicey time, because as the husband's patience starts running out he may drop a libido-crushing bomb that will agitate you so completely you could almost cry. It might be sulking for sex, asking for a consolation blow job, whining about how tough it is to wait, commenting on how your body has changed, or workout tips on how to get your body back. His desperation blinds him to the fact that one misplaced comment could shatter his progress and add months to the sex drought. Ideally, we would all be stable enough to converse reasonably about these matters, but it rarely pans out that way. We wouldn't recommend this kind of chat unless you have at least a three-hour stretch of sleep between feedings under your belt.

STAYING ON COURSE

Studies say the most common time for male infidelity is within the first six months of his wife giving birth. Men, this is no excuse for sleeping around, and women, this is a friendly FYI. Rather than being discouraged or threatened by his masturbation, think of it as buying time until you get yourself to a saner and more well-rested state. Be thankful for small favors, and be happy he is cheating on you with his own hand.

BOTTOM LINE

There is no magic number of days or weeks it takes to get back to normal after birth. Six weeks is a best-case scenario, six months may put your relationship in the red zone. Men, help your cause by helping out, and trying to lick your chops discreetly. Women, you have to start somewhere, so saddle up.

WHY YOU SHOULD CARE

Men: You care because six weeks is long enough, but you don't want to put her health or your future sex life at risk. You may feel that you've been patient, with little or no acknowledgment, and that you're long overdue for some good lovin'. Your patience during this journey is an investment that will pay off in the hopefully, not-so-long run.

Women: This may be the first time your sexual desire has waned or come into question. Physically reconnecting with your husband is a priority for the health of your marriage. Finding your way back to your sexual self will help you start feeling human again. Look at these first experiences as an investment in your own libido-recharge program.

WHAT YOU CAN DO

Men: Nothing delays the libido-recharge program more than pressure, sulking, whining, watching the game with a full sink of dishes, or dispensing diet tips. Forget the old trusted tricks for getting her into the sack and understand that the new turn-ons are help and sleep. Change diapers, rock the baby to sleep, do the dishes, and help organize the family life to ease the bitterness. Women don't intend to create a barter-based sex situation, but when a man helps with the general list of to-dos, it speeds her trip back to herself, which ultimately leads to more sex for you. Have we mentioned yet in this chapter to be supportive of her body? Not every man has to sincerely tell his wife she is at her most beautiful when pregnant, nursing, toting pasty jugs, whatever. But DO NOT make her feel worse about her post-science-experiment body, or dwell on the sketchy details about what she looks and feels like down under.

Women: Be aware that even when your mind and body feel ready, the first entry can be brutal, thanks to scar tissue and the Sahara-like dryness in your former oasis. Take the advice of many wise women: grab a handful of K-Y jelly, slap it on there, and give it a go. It still has to be slow and gentle, but it will be the beginning of something. Even if it's comfortable, sex the first few times may not be that excellent. If you feel some pleasure, count yourself lucky and cling to that liferaft all the way back to a healthy sex life. If you don't feel much pleasure, keep at it until you do. Enjoying sex again happens when you can start associating positive feelings with sex, and it takes repeated experiences until the pleasure outweighs the sacrifices. The good news is that technology is making it easier. New lubes like Silk-E and Astroglide come to the rescue. When they say "a little dab will do you," they are not kidding. Developed by a NASA researcher, Astroglide *is* rocket science at its domestic best. Plus it makes excellent, if expensive, bike chain lubricant—slick and sex-life changing!

CHANGES THEY DON'T TELL YOU ABOUT IN BIRTHING CLASS

There are quite a few things they don't tell you in the pregnancy brochures, possibly because of a conspiracy theory to keep this info under raps in the name of preserving the human race. These may seem like "women things," but inasmuch as they affect the way women feel physically and emotionally, they affect sex drive and thus, by definition, become "men things" as well. So read on if you dare to take an uncensored look at the postpartum revisionist geography of the female anatomy.

VAGINA

If you were ever concerned about a nasty odor that emitted from your crotch, nothing can top the horrendous smell of lochia, the post-birth discharge that can last up to six weeks. Be grateful for this handy, built-in repellent as it gives a chance for the bruised and battered war zone to recover and for the weighty swelling to recede. Other treats you may discover are bothersome skin tags, that may or may not have to be removed, and excessive bleeding, which of course should be reported to your doctor.

BREASTS

After the baby is born the milk comes in with a vengeance, making your breasts take on a life of their own. They launch off your chest so fast that they can become huge fleshy heaves covered with purple stretch marks and blue veins coursing down to a nipple the size of your head in a color never before seen on your body. These jugs may not look or feel like erogenous zones to you, and by all means their involvement in your sexual contact is at your discretion, but don't be surprised if your partner wants a piece of them. And beware the aroused nursing breasts—they spray like hydrants.

BLADDER

Bladder control, or lack thereof, is a potentially long-lasting side effect of childbirth. It can keep you in Depends or just at home for fear of "losing it" in public while sprinting, jumping, running, or even standing up. Do yourself a favor and pack some extra undies along with those diapers for the baby. Do your kegel exercises—they will help, we promise.

HEMORRHOIDS

Not everyone gets these delightful wonders, but after the pressure of a baby, stress, and the unrealized need for extra water and fiber, sometimes your backside launches into a post-birth bouquet of hemorrhoids that look like a bunch of grapes. Sit on the baby bop pillow that was meant for resting your nursing baby, get some horizontal time, take in lots of water and fiber, spread on the special creams, work the anal kegels, and trust that the body heals.

EPISIOTOMY

When labor really starts shaking down, you stop caring where and how the baby could possibly make it out. People cringe when they hear about the doctor giving an episiotomy by cutting into the perineum. At that point, the doctor could get out the chainsaw. Progress toward birth is what we are looking for at that stage. Healing after a tear or an episiotomy will involve ice packs and a one-cheek lean.

"I don't care how your relationship worked before kids. After kids, it's tit for tat."

—female, age 38

"There is no question that my sex life improves when I do dishes and keep the kids out of my wife's hair for some time each day."

—male, age 44

Positive Balance: Understanding the Structure of Your Sex Account

There is no doubt that the magnanimous glow of togetherness—the blissful state where our generosity toward each other knows no limits—fades a bit when the reality of getting stuff done in a household intrudes. We eventually ease into our roles, only to have that equitable division of labor totally blown apart with the arrival of kids, and the new tasks heaped upon both partners. What emerges is the accounting feature of relationships, a fluctuating balance of goodwill currency that directly affects even the most robust, mutually satisfying sex lives.

MONITORING THE ACCOUNT

Your account balance, while directly related to your sex life, is not about earning or owing sex. Rather, it is a measure of the acknowledgment, appreciation, and respect each party feels toward the other. Making ample deposits and reasonable withdrawals allows your partner to feel good about wanting to satisfy you. Likewise, if you're always depleting the account, you gradually lose the ability to earn interest and ultimately have no goodwill credit on which to draw. At this point, you may notice communications become terse and your sex life is not that great. As far as who monitors the account, that duty falls to, as one woman explains, "Whoever is getting the shaft and doing more than their share at the moment."

Often that would be women, either in their traditional roles of stay-at-home moms on duty 24/7, or as full-time working parents who still feel they bear the responsibility of being the primary caregiver. Women often have a hard time relinquishing household control or asking their men to step up to the sink.

Contrary to widely accepted stereotypes, there are certain math concepts that women can calculate in their heads faster than a Pentium processor. She may use this skill when weighing the caloric options of a glass of wine versus a slice of birthday cake in the context of the length and intensity of her morning run, factoring in the number of days until she has to get into a bathing suit. She also uses it to keep track of your "personal" checking and savings accounts. Without pen, paper, or comment she can monitor multiple floating balances with remarkable accuracy.

ACCOUNT ACTIVITY

Non-earning parents, who often feel like they "owe" for being a "kept" spouse, achieve positive balance by shouldering all the day-to-day child-care and household duties, an unpaid job, which, for anyone who has fully experienced it can agree, is full-time, esteem-busting, and largely thankless. But that's part of the deal. What's not part of the deal is the lingering anachronism that the female's role of primary domestic responsibility extends beyond the workday to every waking moment. Indeed, that relentless Groundhog Day–scenario spawned the necessity for "mommy's little helpers" like cocktail hour, diet pills, chocolate truffles, and therapy. In this post–June Cleaver era, with activities and responsibilities for both spouses that lie well beyond the home, it is expected that during non-work hours and on weekends both parents are equally on duty. Of course, it never works neatly that way, so at any one time one partner is always shouldering more of the burden, while the other, ideally, picks up the slack. When that doesn't happen, resentment ensues, which, if not expressed and resolved, gets reconciled in the account.

Consider this scene that transpired between a husband and wife, a nice normal couple with a healthy relationship, that is nonetheless account driven: The soft-spoken woman, rushing out the door at 7:30 a.m. to drop kids at school and then go to work, yells back to her husband, who is reading the paper before he ambles to work alone an hour later, "Just do the goddamned dishes in the sink before you go!"

The man is momentarily surprised at her outburst, and may not immediately make the connection between sex and doing the dishes. To the many men who claim that they know nothing about the existence and operations of the sex account, here's how it works in this example. Certainly, at 7:30 a.m., doing the stack of dishes from the night before—a chore he apparently neglects on occasion—is not going to get him laid any time soon. But not doing the dishes is going to drive his account down and, combined with similar transgressions, make sex a very remote possibility in the near term. Doing these dishes now will keep him from plunging further into the red, while doing the dishes unbidden (and the night before) the next time will steadily contribute to building his account.

When you're banking on sex, there are really two accounts at work: the checking account that funds your immediate sex needs and the savings account that represents the value of your long-term assets. You need to pay attention to both. Here's an example of a man relying solely on his checking account with no regard for his savings account. Just before bedtime he meticulously tends to his wife's foreseeable needs. He dims the lights, turns down the bed, puts her book on her bedside table, turns on the electric blanket, and makes the bed inviting in every way. He's doing all the right things to facilitate his immediate sexual needs being met. But in his wife's mind: "It makes me think. If he can do all that why can't he fix the microwave that has been broken for four months?"

BUILDING LONG-TERM CURRENCY

As stated earlier, maintaining accounts is all about respect, and it pays to keep that longer-term goal in mind, as illustrated by this 38-year-old mother of an infant and toddler, with no libido in sight:

"When we have not had sex in a while my husband is edgy, irritable, and uncomfortable with himself in a low-self-esteem kind of way. He doesn't push and he doesn't beg; he is totally dignified in the way he respects my feelings or lack of drive. So sometimes, I feel like taking one for the team because I know he will feel better, he will think more clearly, and will be much more pleasant to be around for the upcoming week. Plus, his physical relief allows him to do better at his job (in sales), which means bigger commissions which is good for both of us! Granted, that's more of a perk than a motivator."

The key to making these accounts work for you is to recognize the symbiotic nature of an intimate relationship. Put crassly, you're using each other. You need each other, if not actually to survive, then certainly to thrive. And you will thrive by maintaining mutual respect. It's about pulling your part of the load to show you are on the same team. "Resentment is a terrible dose of icy water on the libido," says one woman. "If my husband is more helpful, more available to support me, I am much more interested in making him happy."

GIVING CREDIT WHERE CREDIT IS DUE

Women, whether they are taking care of the kids exclusively or working outside the home, need to recognize the value of their husbands' contributions and show their gratitude as well. One youngish buck complained: "I work all day, bring her flowers, do all the dishes at night, and try to make her feel good about herself. And I still feel like I am 'stealing' sex. How much more am I supposed to do?"

One salesman who predicted a frigid homecoming reception from his boys' trip grumbled, "She's going to make me pay. And if I even touch her in bed she's going to be mad that I want sex. I'd rather just roll over than deal with all that." Bringing home the bacon is no small task, nor is coaching soccer, tackling the "honey-do" list, and other things women often expect men just to do in their free time. Sex therapists report that women, in particular, deny sex as a form of punishment or to shift the balance of power to their favor. We all need down time and we all want to get full credit for what we bring to the table. While women are more likely to monitor the accounts, men can make the accounts work for them by understanding the basics of what moves the balance from black to red.

THE FLOW OF FUNDS

Most shifts in the balance are predictable. He does the dishes, takes out the garbage, makes the kids lunches, lets you sleep in every now and then, or remembers important dates and occasions—his balance goes up. He forgets to pick up the kids at school, doesn't tell you he's going out with the guys on book club night, or gives you a vacuum cleaner for Christmas—his balance goes down. His boys' night turned into a weekend and he comes home hungover with a duffel of dirty laundry: his remaining balance is automatically zeroed out.

She expresses appreciation for his efforts to help around the house, allows him time with the boys without comment, backs up his parenting style, or takes care to make sex a priority—her balance goes up. She spends hours on the phone, overdips on self-indulgences, puts friends ahead of him, or ditches him for hours with the kids—her balance goes down. She brutally shuts him down, withholds sex, or compares him to an old boyfriend: her remaining balance is zeroed out. The fact that your account can be zeroed out—up or down—in one act/service/situation/transgression can work for or against you. Everyone has a different value system, so you're well advised to understand your partner's system and exploit it to your benefit.

BONUS TERRITORY

Here's where your opportunity lies. By being thoughtful and helpful you are proactively building your balance. This can be through impulsive acts, such as planning a weekend away, that boost your checking account, or long-term positive shifts of behavior that compound interest in your savings. Attention to what really makes your partner happy is what puts you in bonus territory. That can mean merely granting periods of freedom for your partner to pursue a purely selfish interest, of temporary freedom from responsibility. The woman who lets her husband golf on Mother's Day, when the links are empty, gets bonus points. The man who surprises his wife by taking the kids and sending her to get a massage gets bonus points. The very act of good sex can be its own bonus. According to one Type A hyper-organized woman who needs everything in its place to be happy, "When we have satisfying sex it puts me in such a good zone that I don't care if he leaves the cupboards open and the cereal box out. It's like an insurance policy for him. Whatever he does or doesn't do for a while is okay."

WHAT DO *WE* KNOW?

Cindy: "When my husband and I were first married we gravitated to the household tasks we did best: I did laundry, and he did dusting and vacuuming; I took beds, he took bathrooms; and I filled the woodbox because getting ahead gives my psyche a serious boost. When we became innkeepers, our physical labor multiplied. Initially, we stuck with the same things, but now that Bruce recognizes that slaying dragons off our list is an investment in creating more free time and head space for both of us, he took over the woodbox. Suddenly, he is ahead in the account system, and I am on the slacker side of things."

Edie: "We all really want to be above the accounting thing, and not turn into one of those couples that exists in a cycle of nagging and drudgery. But family life—particularly in the baby-raising phase—can make you snap. I know perfectly normal women who counted the number of diapers they changed in comparison to their husbands, and who tallied up the hours of alone time each spouse was getting per week. It's crazy. When hunkered in the trenches we need to understand we are working in a compromised en-

THE FINE PRINT: WHAT DOESN'T COUNT

Men take note—wait to get your strokes in the sack. If you angle for affirmation for any of these helpful deeds, duties, and gestures, or if you take them on heroically then feign incompetence to get rescued, they don't count. One woman recalls her husband's offer to make dinner after she had a particularly harrowing day. He rummaged around the fully stocked gourmet kitchen for a while and finally emerged to ask, "Where do we keep the fresh crab?" Doesn't count.

Women take note—playing the martyr sucks all the gratitude from the recipient of your "toils." Slaving over his favorite dinner, then dropping it in front of him in a sweaty huff doesn't count.

A goodwill gesture doesn't count if: you have to be asked to do it; you whine or complain about it; you need to be reminded of basic household tasks when on duty (every adult in the house should know what day is garbage day); you do something great like bring home takeout for dinner but don't tell her first (a little communication can save your ass!); you over-dramatize the execution of the task; you "happen" to mention the hardship you endured to complete the task; or you make the receiving party feel guilty in any way.

DAILY FLUCTUATIONS

The account doesn't have to be reconciled daily, and certainly an important part of a good relationship is keeping the bigger picture of each other's roles and contributions in view. The whole "for richer or poorer, in sickness and in health" thing speaks to a certain amount of slack we should cut each other. Nonetheless, it is wise to monitor our accounts

vironment and we have to be vigilant about finding out and then helping deliver what each other values. An expensive dinner out might be worth nothing while three hours to go on a bike ride is priceless."

BOTTOM LINE

Whether you know it or not, there likely is an accounting system in place in your relationship and whoever is on the losing end of the equation (that is, pulling more of the load), is monitoring the account. You can decry or deny it—or you can understand it, embrace it, and make it work for you.

WHY YOU SHOULD CARE

You'll have more sex and better sex by staying out of the red zone. Little things can keep you in the black. Building goodwill isn't about the big stuff.

closely enough to have a sense of whether we are safely cushioned in the black, hovering in balance, or plunging into the red zone. The easiest way to do this is by agreeing on our mutual expectations beforehand. Without those parameters, it's all too easy to let the balance get way out of control and then release the tension by snipping, biting, or exploding.

BEWARE THE WINDFALLS

As investment advisors say, if it seems too good to be true, it probably is. One 37-year-old father of three young kids could not believe his good fortune when, while lying next to his wife in bed, she offered up a blow job. "I thought I would do the noble thing and say, 'No, honey let's make love.' But I didn't have the willpower and blurted 'yes, yes, yes.'" Two weeks after that when he brought up the prospect of sex, she slapped him with the bankbook. "Are you kidding? What about that blow job I gave you. Can't that hold you over?"

LIMITED LIABILITY CLAUSE

Neither of you is responsible for past accounts. You are not responsible for filling any emotional void that may stem from your partner's past. "We acknowledge the things we need because of our pasts, even though they may be unrelated to our own past together," says one couple. Men, don't expect a woman to be the mother you never got enough care from, as well as your lover. Sorry, but this is especially true during cold and flu season when women manage to stay upright. Women, don't expect a man to be a tender confidante who also wants to ravage you. You need both, but that's why you have girlfriends. Use them to fill some of the tenderness void so you're not so needy.

Remember that, as in other areas of the relationship, your partner is not psychic. Speaking in code, or not speaking at all, does nothing to improve your balance.

WHAT YOU CAN DO

Men: Staying even is a dynamic process, not just a matter of keeping your nose clean. Do yourself a huge favor and remember the everyday basics, like appreciation. The man who brings home major bucks, pays for a housekeeper, and makes sure all his wife's needs are met on a macro level still needs to show his wife appreciation in little personal ways to maintain the day-to-day balance of his checking account. As one woman notes, "He needs a friendly 'hello' and 'goodbye' when entering and leaving the house.

I need acknowledgment of gratitude when I put food on the table. I don't need him sitting there like a fifth child." You can lose a lot of credit by forgetting occasions like your anniversary, her birthday, Valentine's Day, and Mother's Day. These aren't important for all women, but you know by now if it's important to your partner. It takes very little on these occasions either to score big or to blow it.

Exploit and explore your bonus territory. Plan escapes for each other, do things without being reminded, express gratitude for everyday things, organize a kid event, arrange a break when she's on duty, plan nights out and do everything from making the reservation to getting the babysitter. Surrender to the full reality of a task without needing to get rescued. You get bonus points for pretty much anything that takes stuff off her shoulders because it not only helps her, but also shows appreciation for what she usually does.

And don't forget to invest in the future. It's always wise to stockpile goodwill. Men who take on baby duties from the very beginning may not be getting any action for those first six weeks, but the break they are giving their wives—especially considering that it is not in exchange for immediate sex—goes straight into the savings account. These men are not only more connected with their kids, but also more attractive to their wives.

Women: Be clear and not resentful. Resentment is the unseen charge that eats at your account. If he's not understanding the source of your displeasure he needs to be told, by you, in words—not sighs, gestures, and snotty Post-its.

Give men a way to build up their accounts. Let them know what part of the load you expect them to share, then let them fly on their own without micromanaging. If it's in their best interest, they make it work. "When my husband wants to escape with the older kids and take them skiing, he finds a way to remember all their gear. And if he forgets something critical, he only does it once." Loosen the reins, let go, and enjoy, instead of complaining that you shoulder the whole load. When they are gone and you truly get a break you look forward to them coming home.

At the same time, be realistic and know that we all play the same game. "When he needs to have sex, he pays a lot of attention and does nice things around the house. The day after he's focused on his own stuff. It makes me mad, but to some extent it makes sense. I'm the same way when I want a new bicycle."

♀ ♂

"My husband had just finished folding laundry after the kids were in bed one night and he suggested we have sex. When I didn't jump on the offer immediately he said, 'What about those two baskets of foreplay over there?' How could I resist that?"
—female, age 37

"I would sooner cancel our cable than our housecleaner. She's not very good, but when my wife wants to save money and get rid of the housecleaner I remind her how we used to wake up every Saturday and scramble to clean the house from top to bottom. That's no way to spend your free time together."
—male, age 43

The Little Things Can Get You Laid

Our culture has trained us to view sex as a spontaneous act, and certainly when you don't have a job or kids and you are freshly infatuated, it is. But that dreamworld is necessarily short-lived. One byproduct of committing to career and relationships is the indispensable role of planning. In adult life as most working people know it, fulfilling your sexual desires is more about steady progress than spontaneity, so you have to look ahead and plan your moves.

THE FOREPLAY OF FOREPLAY

Even when both partners have the desire and intent for sex on a given evening, there are things that can throw you off track throughout the day. Men need to be especially mindful of this because women report that their desire can easily be derailed by the slightest obstacle. Conversely, everyone has specific things that can move him or her toward the possibility of sex. If you are in a long-term relationship these little productivity turn-ons and domestic niceties—the Foreplay of Foreplay—are just as likely to get you laid as chocolate, lingerie, and a Swedish massage. The willingness of your partner for sex on any given night might begin at 8 a.m. in a wide variety of forms.

THE BACKFIRE OF DESIRE

Considering the physical effects of bearing children, not to mention the libido-numbing general monotony of family life and the nearly standard difference of sex drive between men and women, couples seeking a healthy sex life have a challenging task. Women feel alternatively guilty for being uninterested in having lots of sex, and bitter about the desperation they hear—or more often feel—from the other side of the bed. Those conflicting emotions, which can flip like a switch, often lead women to passive-aggressive defensive strategies such as flossing their teeth excessively, busying themselves with kitchen tasks, or checking email until their husbands fall asleep. Meanwhile, the man in this situation feels more frustrated and denied, and physically or verbally grasps at any prospect of sex he can, hoping for a miraculous turnover. This perceived aggression in turn typically pisses the woman off even more, which can lead couples to the point where communicating about sex openly is no longer possible. It can become an explosive situation, figuratively and literally, due to the condition of pent-up fluids commonly referred to as DSB (Deadly Sperm Buildup).

Men who to want to avoid DSB and women who want to avoid causing it need to recognize what kinds of things have to align to get them on the path toward sex. Getting into a sexual frame of mind sometimes requires crossing a figurative bridge. This bridge bypasses the many obstacles that can pop up along the road and rattle her libido into a ditch. Each woman is enticed across The Bridge by a different combination of factors. However, The Bridge may easily collapse if she harbors unaddressed resentment.

WHAT DO WE KNOW?

Cindy: "Being in a relationship for six years before we got married gave Bruce and me the opportunity to experience the uncensored disparity in the sex drive department. The low point in our connection came a few years into our relationship, when Bruce traveled a lot as a ski coach. His job, while it included world travel and interesting people, was more physically exhausting and emotionally draining than glamorous. Bruce usually returned home with little work to do, a lot of time on his hands, and a hearty appetite for sex.

"I missed him as well, and certainly still loved him, but his rabid desire for sex chafed me and was starting to drive me away to the point where I avoided cuddling with him or doing anything that would get him aroused. His reaching out morphed into sulking and desperation while I countered with more avoidance. Neither of us could openly dissect the situation and a wedge grew between us.

"It all blew up for me after a particularly hellish day teaching first grade. I returned home—where I had kept the woodstove burning myself for weeks—anticipating plopping on the couch with Bruce (who had returned from a three-week trip the night before) and a hot cup of tea in our cozy little house.

"My happiness about his return instantly drained when I walked into the house. There he sat, huddled under a few extra layers of fleece because he had let the fire go out—and angling for sex. He could not have found a more instant way to douse my desire. Now, if he had kept the fire going all day, would I have been running upstairs stripping my clothes off with gusto as I went? Doubtful, but the fire situation triggered a backload of penalties, while keeping it going would have actually helped set the wheels in motion. Keeping systems going and maintaining efficiency happen to be contributing factors to my sex drive."

> "Watching a man doing housework is one of the sexiest activities I know. I'd prefer it to Swedish porn any day. Fewer pole dancing classes for women and more ironing lessons for men is what I say."
> —Carol Hunt
> The Sunday Independent
> (Ireland)

Edie: Timing is everything. When it's an especially busy witching hour—dinner is cooking, kids need to be marshaled inside and bathed, homework done, lunches packed, piano practiced, etc, etc, etc. I feel like an overextended juggler in a bad circus act. If, at that moment, my husband comes home and starts tidying up, instead of tending to one of my many immediate needs with getting things under control, I get really pissy, and no matter where I was before that moment, The Bridge has now been bombed. Now, as with many women, I create this scenario. It's not that I want to do all those things with no help, but I want to be the kind of person who can handle it all, so I neglect to delegate until it's too late and I'm in over my head. If I told him calmly, well in advance, of the kind of help I need (and don't need) in this situation, he would gladly give it. I think a lot of couples need to meet in the middle—the women need to be a lot more forthcoming and the men need to be a bit more perceptive.

EASING THE LOAD

With so many landmines in a woman's path toward sex, men are well-advised to act as minesweepers by removing household tasks and stresses whenever and wherever possible. These are different for every woman, so it's a process of trial and error to see what actions make the biggest difference. The negative effects of not helping out are all too familiar to women who are often mired in domestic drudgery, as described by this 40-year-old working mom with young children: "The times I least want to have sex are when I feel like an old-fashioned housewife who does every menial thing for the family. After a day of slaving, then cooking, serving, and cleaning up dinner . . . when we get in bed and his hand comes over, I hate him. I really do, for not realizing how little I want to put out energy for another person."

Doing the dishes, feeding the kids dinner, or helping with homework can be a slam dunk for some men, but not quite enough for others. One 43-year-old man honing his recipe for success notes that, "Flowers do not work, vacuuming helps more. Being on time goes a long way, as does asking her opinion, letting her choose the TV show, and not making her watch sports. Talking about what she did or wants to do, and listening to what the kids say or do probably gets me the most mileage."

Some women actually have a negative reaction to housekeeping help, if they interpret it as a sign of their inadequacy. One woman finds herself wracked by guilt when her husband takes on household chores for which she has not solicited his help: "If my husband slaves away cleaning things up, or folding the eight loads of laundry kicking around the bedroom, I feel horribly guilty about what a terrible wife and housekeeper I am. I cannot stop myself from thanking him profusely while at the same time apologizing and asking if he's angry at me even if he isn't. If he does a few things it doesn't press my guilt button, but doing a major effort has me cringing!"

A way around this potential roadblock is paying people to do your dirty work. One woman was surprised by the positive effect of hiring a weekly cleaning service. "I had no idea how much it was weighing on me—the dread of cleaning and the guilt of not cleaning—until it was off my plate." Many couples find that hiring out tasks helps them connect not only by easing the general stress level and workload, but by acknowledging that they'd rather spend time together than fight over who is going to scrub the toilets and fix the broken fence.

MORNING NOONER NIGHT?

Merging your paths toward sex can be as simple as finding the time when you are both mentally and physically primed for sex. The association of sex with bedtime doesn't work well when couples are exhausted after a full day of work and parenting. Add to that a belly full of dinner and perhaps a glass of wine, and even our lustiest intentions can fade. "By 9 p.m. I am beat," says one woman. "Morning is where it's at for me." Physically, that might be ideal for men, whose testosterone levels typically peak at 8 a.m. While that is a completely inconvenient time for most working people and families, the early shift in general is a time when many people feel uncluttered, refreshed, and mentally clear for sex. One woman who is an advocate for morning action says, "I love the morning. You're not tired, you can get showered right then, and start the day right."

The nooner fantasy is out of reach for most people for all sorts of reasons, even on weekends, because daylight presents an endless supply of tasks that need to be tended. But nooners can put a spring in your step if circumstances allow, and also blaze the path toward more sex later in the day as one woman reported, "The kids were in school and my husband happened to be home so we had afternoon sex. We both were so turned on that we couldn't wait to have sex that night and again the next morning before he went to work."

SETBACKS

One couple who has the coveted educator's schedule—weekends, vacations, and summers free together—keeps an admirably healthy pace during their time off. While both are satisfied and comfortable with their sex life, the ongoing effort to "close the deal" even during times when they are both on vacation can cause low-grade tension at times. She likes the idea of planning sex, but it doesn't always work because she wants the option to change her mind if she is exhausted or "not psyched for sex" by nighttime.

He describes that she is not a moody person, but she is like a "sex seismograph," responding to tremors throughout the day. An unpleasant phone call with one of her parents, a change of mood because of an interaction with the kids, or a story on the news about something violent—anything can tip the scale. "Sometimes we are on the road to having sex as the evening approaches. I have done the dishes, packed the lunches, and given her a foot rub while we watch a movie. Then the story shifts in the movie and it's all over."

He is so tuned in to her reactions that he admits to trying to keep her in a news-protected bubble, letting her know if she should read the paper each day. "It's not only because it will decrease his chances to have sex," she says, "but also because he knows that anything sad or harsh may affect me for days. He screens movies for me in case it will put me in a funk. I know it sounds pathetic, but it's true."

Often a seemingly minor action can pack enough meaning to trigger a major reaction. One woman describes how the act of shutting the door makes her shut down. "We never close our bedroom door, so when he closes the door before coming to bed it shows me he assumes he is going to get some, whether or not I am game. The fact that he is assuming it's a done deal that we are having sex that night immediately pushes my buttons and I shut him down on principle."

> "When you're wrong apologize to her in front of a lot of people. Major points."
> —male, age 32

Some things are simply deal killers, as described by one women who insists men should never wake women up to have sex. "I fail to find it amusing to wake up in the morning with a penis being jammed into my backside with little nudges. A few more minutes of sleep when you are tired is better than any orgasm you can have."

PRESS PAUSE

Reinforcing the genuine desire for connection is perhaps the most universally appreciated act. Little kindnesses work wonders when they reflect deep feelings of respect.

> "Take a moment out of your busy schedule, regardless of everything that is going on in your life, and spend time connecting with your spouse. We have date night every week, and we share responsibility for it. Each of us is responsible for planning two Saturday nights a month. It keeps things fresh and neither person gets stuck doing all the planning. It also allows us to talk about 'the little things' we can do to help each other—and ultimately gets us back in the sack."
> —male, age 43

BOTTOM LINE

The desire for sex is a buildup of scenes rather than an impromptu performance. Setting the stage with little acts of respect and kindness will earn you an encore.

WHY YOU SHOULD CARE

Men: Knowing what little things you can do to put her in the mindset, and showing a genuine effort to make those things happen, gives you more power over the outcome. When the time comes, you'll not only have sex, but it'll be present-and-accounted-for sex, instead of that preoccupied "I have to remember to pick up the dry cleaning" sex.

Women: Knowing and communicating these little things that help clear your agenda for sex will fairly shore up his odds, lighten your load, and disentangle your sexual-desire issues from your general-household-chore-disgruntlement issues.

WHAT YOU CAN DO

Men: Invest time and energy into figuring out what it is that gets her across The Bridge with patience. Try to distinguish what would make her life less stressful by taking on tasks around the house or with the kids that will clear her plate.

Women: Give him points for trying, even if he misses a bit on delivery. If your man makes the effort to tune into what helps your daily life, he deserves some genuine positive reinforcement. Instead of fixating on unmet needs and expectations, tell him what stands between you and The Bridge.

> *"I think the best way to show love is in the everyday little things you do for each other. One time I was leaving on a trip and before I went I made sure to go into the garden and pick some of her favorite flowers and put them in a vase. When she saw them she made some comment about it being the wrong vase. By the time I got to the airport she had called to basically tell me she was an idiot."*
> —male, age 55

♀	♂
"My husband gets offended when I say this, but I look at sex sort of like a cookie. If I have it I really like it, and if not I don't miss it." —female, age 43	*"I get that most women are less horny than most men, but that doesn't mean it is right."* —male, age 44

✳ Drive Differential ✳

We go into our relationships with fairly equitable sex drives fueled by raw attraction. There is even a word for this insatiable feeling that sucks us into thinking monogamy will be easy. The passionate intensity of a new romantic relationship is called "limerance." It has a nice ring to it, sort of a cross between a poem and a trance.

Limerance is what makes us want to devour each other like raw cookie dough at every opportunity, what makes us envision a future together of intense romance built on deep physical and emotional connection. During limerance, both partners produce phenylethylamine, a natural amphetamine known as the "chemical of love." Sadly, we get over it—both the love meds and limerance fade. Sadder still, we get over it at differing rates. And when we get over it, we revert to our natural sex drives, which we express and prioritize differently.

The difference in desire for sex between men and women is common—books are written about it, counselors survive on it, marriages break up over it—and yet it remains an unspoken point of contention. As if we didn't know this already from personal experience, the topic has been aggressively studied ever since Alfred Kinsey's *Sexual Behavior in the Human Male,* and later *Sexual Behavior in the Human Female* brought the private domain public, and primed the sex-info-starved public for William Masters' and Virginia Johnson's studies that took sexology into the lab. Masters' and Johnson's *Human Sexual Response* was derived from their work of observing and measuring the physical responses of 700 men and women during masturbation and intercourse. It defined the sexual response cycle as we know it today. The book came out in 1966, immediately and perhaps not coincidentally just before 1967's "summer of love," which propelled the quest for good lovin' into an open forum. And yet, despite the ensuing tidal wave of studies and surveys that swamp us with stats and advice, we find ourselves faced with the same old problem: While erection and orgasm problems can be diagnosed like engine trouble, desire is a mysterious starter that won't turn over.

DRIVER'S EDUCATION

"Men are like firefighters. The boots and trousers are lined up, pointed in the right direction. You're ready to slide down that pole. Sometimes the alarm goes off, but it's a false alarm. Sorry Sparky, boots on, nowhere to go." —male, age 52

As one woman's husband told her, "You don't know how much men think about sex. All day long!" According to neuropsychiatrist Louann Brizendine in *The Female Brain*, 85 percent of men between the ages of 20 and 30 think about sex every 52 seconds, while women think about it once a day, or up to three or four times on their most fertile days. Furthermore, studies find that in long-term relationships male desire stays constant while the female's motivation decreases steadily after a couple of years in a relationship. Even if a woman is receptive to maintaining the limerance levels of sex she is less likely to be proactive. As one 50-year-old man on his second marriage wonders: "What is it about putting that ring on the finger? Once you get married, the sex is over. Why does that make women change the deal?"

Even though some men see it that way, it's not that simple or that instant. At times it feels that one of Mother Nature's cruelest little jokes is the mismatch of male and female sex drive. Crueler still is how we never see it coming until we are in the rat's nest of work and parenting

"A happy man is a drained man." —female, age 46

with neither the time nor perspective to deal with our sexual dissatisfaction. At a time of life when many women could be savoring their physiological sexual peaks they are instead fumbling in a cloud of colliding forces: Bitterness at unequal parenting roles, or the pressure to have more, better sex; fatigue of juggling work, family, and social obligations; guilt about not staying home or not working or doing both but not well enough. On top of all of this, add lack of privacy and the length of time it takes for women to orgasm, and you'll start to see why a woman's relative lack of desire is really a simple matter of time (or lack thereof). Says one working, 36-year-old mother of two: "I tell my husband, 'Fifteen minutes. That's all you've got. If it's going to be 20 that's not going to work for me.'" Many women in the trenches of childrearing simply don't see the orgasm payoff to be worth the time investment.

None of this factors into the sex decision for the single woman; it piles up as her relationship progresses into long-term cohabitation and then parenting. So yes, the deal changes, but it changes for both partners. While most women wouldn't trade the benefits of motherhood for all our former liberties, this stage of life carries unavoidable burdens that shift our priorities progressively away from our own gratification. It may be Mother Nature's way of protecting both partners from more than we can take on.

"My latest reverse psychology is to tell him how excited I am about the idea of having another baby. I spread my legs and get a big smile on my face pretending to be ready and willing. He immediately crawls back to his side of the bed for at least another week. It works way better than the 'I have a headache' or 'I'm too tired' excuses."
—female, age 36

CROSSING THE BRIDGE

Men take note, when it comes to dealing with rejection, women can't relate. One woman thinks back and estimates she's been shut down three times in 15 years. Guys often take women's relative lack of interest personally, as a sign of rejection, while women feel they either have to defend or apologize for their flagging interest. The rejection and resentment cycle leads to less sex, less connection, and less mutual desire, which spirals right down to less sex again.

The obstacles to sex are for most, painfully familiar. Making sex a priority for a woman with kids, amidst obligations to work, family, and community, as well as the need for sleep and maybe some exercise, is a multi-step effort. Getting yourself and your partner into the mindset is the first step. Once you have decided it would be good for you to have sex, then you have to find the time and the way to get each other across The Bridge from apathy to appetite.

Men are usually willing to do anything to help this process, even though they don't have a personal frame of reference for it. For most women, sex is an affirmation for all that's good in a relationship, and follows as a consequence of connection. Sex plays a different role in the male psyche. Men are more apt to attribute sex to a McGuyver-like power to fix anything that ails a relationship and to fuse whatever connection is missing. When men feel mad, resentful, or stressed, most report that sex is not only still on their radar, but that it is often their solution to a negative mindset. It seems to relieve stress, get them back their personal and professional mojo, and give them energy and focus. Meanwhile, her own stress and anger do nothing to entice a woman toward intimacy, and in fact pretty much guarantee the chilly roll to the other side of the bed.

One couple's fiery sexual encounter highlights how impossible it is to divert men once they are on The Bridge. The husband worked hard to create a romantic atmosphere with several candles around the bedroom. It was going so well that a wild fling of a limb knocked a candle off the side table. A pillowcase caught on fire. Coitus was interrupted while the two naked firefighters scrambled to smother the fire before it spread and then collapsed in relief among the splattered wax and singed pillowcases. Adrenaline pumping with the vision of burning down their house, sex was the furthest thing from her mind. He immediately rebounded with, "Now where were we?"

GET IT WHILE YOU CAN

Not to complicate sexual desire with buzz-killing statistics, but the reality is that prostate cancer is the second-most-common cancer in men, afflicting one in every six men in their lifetimes. Twenty percent of those having prostate surgery will become permanently impotent, incontinent, or both. In the somewhat joking words of one doctor, "My wife had better take advantage of the mighty Sequoia while it is still straight and tall!"

Despite the stereotype that all men have an insatiable desire for sex, some medical conditions and medications affect erectile function

"Occasionally I remind my wife that she should take advantage of me now while I still have it because I won't always have this drive and you just never know when it may be snatched away."
—male, age 42

and sexual desire in men. In general, about 52 percent of men between the age of 40 and 70 suffer erectile dysfunction. Most of them are over the age of 65, so prevalence increases with age.* Premature ejaculation, for instance, is one of the most common sex inhibitors for men. Even when the condition has been treated, some men may continue to feel anxious about their performance, leading them to shun intimacy.**

> "My husband's medications affect his sex drive. He's only interested in sex about once a month, whereas I desire sex at least once a week. He isn't comfortable addressing the situation, even with me."
> —female, age 44

An increasing number of men suffer from low libido, yet there are few opportunities and very little cultural support to share this with others outside the doctor's office.

Despite the depressing data and anecdotes, a couple's sex drive trajectory can be coaxed to intersect. It takes understanding and communication to recalibrate and stabilize your sex life. In particular, it may be helpful to consider one key factor in the sex drive equation that is rarely mentioned and does not lend itself to blame, guilt, or resentment; namely, the sheer exhaustion caused by just one female orgasm, much less two or three or four, is enough to account for a serious gender discrepancy in the quest for sex.

NASCAR NATION MEETS MAJOR LEAGUE PITCHING

Penis Envy theories notwithstanding, far more men say they covet the pleasure achieved by their women than the other way around. Toting a clitoris is a gift from the creators. That said, it's darned tiring. The act of having sex takes energy—for a man it is roughly the equivalent of walking up two flights of stairs—albeit two long, steep flights of stairs. For a woman it's more like taking ten flights of stairs, at varying speeds from a crawl to an all-out sprint.

The path of the female orgasm and the path of the male orgasm are two entirely different stories. While both have rising action, climax, and a resolution, the plots vary wildly for women. The male orgasm only varies a bit in intensity but generally follows the same path each time, not unlike a NASCAR race. He gets going, and takes a few laps that build speed and power until he bursts through the finish. Then the car gets sent back to

* "Sex Reduces Heart Attack Risk," *Business World,* November 2004
** "Trouble Looms When Couples Lose That Loving Feeling," *2003 Tallahassee Democrat*

the pit crew for new tires, fuel, and fluids, and he is ready to get back on the track when summoned. Regardless of the car model, the entire process doesn't usually take very long.

Sex for women is more like watching baseball. Sometimes there is a lot of action on the field, and sometimes there's not a lot going on. In the middle of the game you might lose interest, be ready to wrap it up, or even have a shopping list going through your head. You get yourself settled after the seventh inning stretch and suddenly, out of nowhere, the bases are loaded. Big Papi steps up to the plate, and this is where it could really go either way. Sometimes you miss the opportunity and muddle through two more innings to end the game, and sometimes, kerplow! It's a grand slam.

Having a clitoris is like being a major league pitcher. After a big night, the pitching arm needs a couple of nights off before it comes back to its full pitching power. For women with kids, sex every day would feel like work without the paycheck. The guilt for not keeping up with demand, as well as the accompanying rejection men feel, is based on unrealistic expectations. Finding a happy medium by making an effort for regular sex, however, will help create a habit that is both physically and emotionally rewarding. Women, turn on your best power of positive thinking for this one and play your open communication card—even if it's the last one for the decade—and it'll be worth it. Having orgasms will help you jog back to the pitching mound. Sure they add to the exhaustion, but they remind you why you started playing the game in the first place.

WHAT DO *WE* KNOW?

Edie: "Given the behavior of some men, I used to assume that their need for sex must be like that desperate urge to pee. Women, you've been there, when you feel like you are going to explode if you can't get to a bathroom quickly: you're eyes are watering, you can't think clearly, you snap at your kids, push people out of your way, and will throw a $20 bill for a two-day old sandwich at the deli to use the 'customers only' restroom. Only that level of intensity can explain some of the behavior we see and hear about from men. But one sporadically sex-starved guy enlightened me with a better analogy. His wife was weaning their infant and the pressure in her breasts had become nearly unbearable. 'I heard her whining about how she needed the baby to suck some of the milk out to relieve the pressure and it hit me. That is exactly how it feels when I haven't had sex for awhile.'"

Cindy: "The tasks involved in running an inn are not that erotic. When our kids are at school, we try to get as much done around the place as we can.

Bruce's fantasy is to have a lot of sex while the kids are at school. It happens maybe four times a year because efficiency and slaying dragons is not only a priority for me, but I just can't become aroused with responsibilities looming.

"One day when we were getting most of our work done ahead of schedule, Bruce seized the opportunity and tempted me to the bed. Well into the event, it suddenly occurred to me that we would need to pick up the tablecloths that afternoon before the guests arrived, and I decided to actually tell him that mid-flight. He managed to maintain his erection through that pathetic moment, and luckily we both had been satisfied by the time the second distraction entered my mind. 'I forgot to buy the green beans while I was at the grocery store!' What a closer. Bottom line for me is that I need to get into a frame of mind before I jump in the sack, no matter how persuasive he can be."

BOTTOM LINE

Men want more, women want some—both have their reasons, ranging from the physical to the emotional. It's the way of the world, not the end of the world.

WHY YOU SHOULD CARE

If you want to keep or make sex a priority, the investment of the woman is really key, because the man rarely requires any convincing to get back in the game. Anger and resentment will not get you closer to your goal, but an honest effort to maintain a healthy relationship will.

WHAT YOU CAN DO

Men: Don't take her lack of interest personally or badger her into having more desire. Shameless pleading usually backfires as well, though with friendly humor it might fly. Work on connecting in non-sexual ways to reinforce that you value the whole relationship, and not merely the service component. To get women on board you need to understand that sexual satisfaction is a more complicated task for women, both emotionally and physically. Once limerance wears off, a positive mindset ignites sexual desire for women. To the men who long for their wives to initiate sex, don't get hung up on the details. Be grateful for the sex you're having. As these two, 43-year-old men advise: "There's no such thing as bad sex. If you're having sex it's good."

Women: You can easily schedule yourself out of sex, but ultimately you are sabotaging your relationship. Making sex a priority is not all about serving his needs but about serving yours as well. Even when you cognitively decide you are ready for sex, sometimes your body won't cooperate because your erogenous zones have been shut down for a while or because your body's sexual desires are overridden by its need for sleep. As mentioned in Getting Back in the Saddle, lube can change the whole experience and be a huge timesaver. The biggest factor, though, is a positive mindset.

One woman attests: "For me sex is like running. I'm not always up for getting up and going out there, but once I'm out, I'm into it and it's enjoyable." Another proposes a less onerous analogy:

"Sex is like yoga. It changes your whole frame of mind every time you do it. It's good for your body, mind, and soul. If we all did yoga a few times a week, life would be better. Why don't we make sex a priority?"

Most women find that crossing The Bridge is worth the journey. How often do you regret a roll in the hay when it's all over?

♀ / ♂

"When we get to seven days with no sex I get no eye contact from him. He sort of looks at me sideways and doesn't talk much." —female, age 39	*"Marriage—especially marriage with kids—is way too much work to enjoy without having an intimate bond (as in frequent sex) with your partner.* —male, age 52

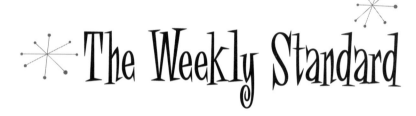

The Weekly Standard

How much sex is normal? When it comes to sex, we want to be within the standard deviation, both for the general population and for each other. The key is finding out what is ideal for each partner, then finding a way to meet in the middle. The more we talk, the more we hear that even when couples want more, they feel within the normal range if they are having sex once a week. "When things are going well . . ." is typically the preface to that answer. But it's a bit like quoting driving times in and around New York City or Los Angeles "without traffic," as if that ideal scenario ever happens. On the highway of everyday life, traffic jams are standard fare.

DIFFERENT FREQUENCIES

Ideal frequency of sex seems to break down more like homeland security codes than hard and fast numbers. At any given moment we are in a zone, and for many couples—even those where both partners aspire to having sex several times per week—the border between green and orange hovers somewhere around a week. That's averaged out over the month, to account for clusters of activity during hormonal surges and no-fly zones around "that time of the month." Our anecdotal evidence is corroborated by the landmark 1994 "Sex in America" study by the University of Chicago that found that Americans have sex about once a week. Given the way everyday life conspires against all ideal scenarios, how do we keep it from drifting into the orange, and how do we know when we are in the red zone or beyond that to the dead zone (see Drought). Is it two weeks? A month?

STANDARD DEVIATION

Young couples, we apologize if this very conversation keeps you from the altar and indeed, it's not the information you hear on the street. Despite strong anecdotal data of realistic expectations, one *Today Show* expert asserted that "only" having sex once a week classifies your marriage as sexless. One woman, who considers she has a healthy sex drive, recently read that the average American married couple has sex 98 times per year. "Who the hell are these people? Don't they have jobs? Kids? A recreational sport?" She admits that family responsibilities suppress her sex life but still, 98 times a year is an average of every 3.72 days, or for those of you with strengths other than math, almost twice a week. Impressive, if true. *Esquire,* in its 2006 "State of the American Man" survey, claims the average man spends 3.2 hours per week having sex. If we allot a generous 30 minutes to each episode, the average guy is getting it more than six times per week. With whom or with what, we wonder, is he having it?

Certainly some couples make the green zone a primary mission and many either aspire to or are in the rhythm of having sex several times per week. One couple in their late 60s claims they have sex every day. God knows we don't want to challenge them for details or proof, but they weathered some rough times in their younger days and this is their vitality. Heck, everyone needs a hobby in retirement.

Even when we snap back to the working world, men are more likely to concur with the TV expert and aspire to the retired couple's ever-green status. "I feel like we (men) get sold a bill of goods," laments one father of three young children, who feels like he married a woman with a healthy sex drive and ended up with a woman who could take or leave sex like a four-day-old blueberry muffin. Indeed, men can relate all too well to the cartoon where a couple is lying in bed and the man is thinking: "Sometimes I fantasize that it's someone else withholding sex from me." Much of that imbalance in expectation may stem from the way men and women communicate among themselves, or not. One woman oberves: "The problem is men don't talk to each other. Women talk, so they know what's in the realm of normal. Men don't know, so they assume everyone is having more sex than they are." Regardless of where men think they fall on the sex meter, they do, in general, want more sex than women.

NATURAL URGES AND ARTIFICIAL EXPECTATIONS

Darwinistically it makes sense. Really, why would a woman's drive be front and center after her procreation window slams shut? Meanwhile, men are in no rush, as demonstrated by Tony Randall and all manner of other golden-aged seed spreaders. Men can shoot live ammo until the day they die, and even longer, though that involves the shocking (literally) use of a cattle prod. Men's sex drives are further fueled by the—largely fantasy-based—assumption that everyone else is having more and better sex, which perpetuates their unrealistically high expectations. One 30-something husband and father of three felt deprived to be having sex "only" two to three times per week. "But then I started talking to other guys and I felt like a porn star."

Such feelings of deprivation are not limited to men middle-aged and older. "They're always tired," remarks one college senior, who takes issue with his girlfriend not wanting sex every time they are together. Before you take it personally, consider all the factors that contribute to a woman's desire for sex that have nothing to do with your prowess and desirability. There is the sheer endurance of the female orgasm as well the time and circumstances it takes to get women into the right mental state, the capriciousness of hormonal fluctuations, and then the real nuts and bolts deterrents to sex, which may include: adding sheets to the already looming pile of laundry, spoiling a perfectly good episode of CSI, having to sleep in the wet spot, wrestling with birth control, waking the kids, and—the aforementioned biggie—losing precious sleep. Many of these factors alone seem inconsequential, but each is enough to let us push sex off another day, and then another.

> "A big part of our breakup had to do with his expectations for sex. He thought we should be having sex every day because, as he said, 'everybody else does.'"
> —divorced female, age 38

MAKING YOUR NUMBERS

Some couples feel like their sex life exists as a running account that needs to be zeroed out at set intervals. One mother who travels periodically for

DOCTORS ORDERS

For couples who are looking for a hard number, Dr. Susan Bennett takes the guesswork out of how much sex we think we should be having, by prescribing her patients a minimum: "I tell my patients they should have sex at least once a week. People need to have sex for their health and their relationships." She explains why we actually do need to have orgasms for optimal health.

"The flaccid penis is anoxic compared to the rest of the body. That means that the oxygen content of penile tissue is low relative to other parts of the body. Regular erections keep the penis well perfused with oxygen-rich blood, avoiding degenerative changes, such as fibrosis." She goes on to explain that the clitoris, if not aroused regularly, can also develop fibrosis, while the vagina gets short, stiff, and very fragile with disuse.

"Without a partner it's hard to keep the vagina healthy. I recommend stretching things out at least once a week—with your fingers if necessary or with a vaginal dialator—particularly in the outer third of the vagina."

work explains she is the accountant in the relationship and maintains positive balance by adhering religiously to the weekly standard. "When I am going to leave for a trip there is so much preparation it is almost more trouble than it's worth. That includes having enough sex to make up for my absence. A guy friend who said he had sex once a week made me kind of step up to that challenge. We've been doing it about two years and it has made our marriage much better. Whether he knows it or not I make sure we don't go beyond a week. It's not like it's in my Palm Pilot, or every Saturday at 9:30 p.m., but I know when I have to go home and have sex with my husband. It's not drudgery, but I'm fulfilling my obligation to maintain the relationship. I can tell when about a week has gone by because my husband gets antsy and whiney and I think, okay, gotta do it. Sometimes it's good. Sometimes it's really good. And sometimes I'm just glad I have a week off again, but in the big scheme it's always worth it."

PENCIL IT IN

Some couples go further and actually plan when they'll have sex. Unromantic as it seems, this is a solid technique. Truthfully, you can't be as spontaneous as you were before kids or as you were early in the relationship when any spare time and any space larger than a locker seemed perfect for sex. One woman first experienced planned sex with her husband by way of offering a dated rain check in a last-ditch effort to buy herself time.

"When the time came we got to it early, and it was really enjoyable. There were no feelings hurt by shutdown or rejection and I thought 'why haven't I thought of that before?'"

Planning can be one-sided too, as it is for the following couple with differing physiological reactions to the act. Sex wakes her up and puts him to sleep. He likes to get in bed early while she usually has work to do at night, but he always manages to wake up for sex. "By the time I went to bed the last thing I wanted to feel was the banana in the back. My win/win solution was to fake going to bed, have sex, then he got his beauty sleep and I was wide awake for a work session."

One couple's decision to boost their sex life by having sex every other day backfired. "That day I felt like a deer in hunting season, and couldn't even walk around in my underwear. Eventually it felt too contrived." You just have to keep adjusting to see what works.

WHAT DO WE KNOW?

Cindy: "People claim that planning ruins the mystery but 'mystery' is a nice euphemism for celibacy. We make a plan in the morning for sex at night and it drives our productivity throughout the day. We both work to clear away the normally late-night tasks and make way for the more enjoyable pursuit."

Edie: "Now that I know entirely too much about everybody else's sex lives, I see that most people care less about exactly how much sex they are having and more about feeling normal. Whether people are having sex once a week or once a month, they want some justification not to feel like a freak about it. Of course the couples who are having the most sex, and are both enjoying it, don't care what anybody else is doing."

BOTTOM LINE

The goal is for both partners to see the benefits of maintaining a minimum balance that is satisfying. You can agree on a reasonable standard either in an actual discussion, or by deductive reasoning that might go something like this: Hmmm, he gets cranky and can't think straight if we haven't had sex in a week, or hmmm she seems a little bitter when I perk up at 2 a.m. and she has to be at work by 7 a.m. There are all kinds of statistics and surveys out there, but each couple has a magic number that works for them. Figure out whatever it is and strive to achieve it.

WHY YOU SHOULD CARE

Men: If you can't get past the fact that you just plain want more, you run the risk of coming across as an ingrate or a whiner. If you strive to reach a balance with her desires you will look like a really sensitive, caring guy, the type of guy women can't help wanting to please, the type of guy who might regularly beat the weekly standard.

Women: Even for those of you who don't desire sex as much as your partner, trust that the desire for sex lives within you as a normal drive. Taking the randomness out of it by making it part of your routine can make it more enjoyable than onerous. Controlling the flow of sex expectations is like putting your mood swings on a metronome. What you can predict you can more easily manage.

WHAT YOU CAN DO

Men: Don't take it personally, or feel like you have to negotiate for sex. Even without the emotional complications of courtship, sex simply takes more effort and energy for most women. This is a partnership in every way, so tune into the times that sex makes sense for you both rather than expecting it every time the urge strikes. Remember, nothing crushes a woman's libido like moping.

Women: If you feel like you're always fighting an imbalance in desire, set a minimum and stick to it. Planning sounds so counter to all the connotations of romance, but it sets you up to get in the mindset. If planning creates a path to "The Bridge," then lay it down. You may surprise yourself and discover the truth of the bumper sticker that reads, "Yield, it's more fun."

"When you lose that connection, you lose the ability to work through other things in your relationship. We didn't break up because of the sex, but if we had been able to keep having sex through the silence of our rough times, I think we would have had a good chance of saving the marriage."
—divorced female, age 56

"What frustrates me is not having enough sex and feeling guilty for asking to have sex. Lying there wondering why she never initiates sex or if we are ever going to have it again or if I should just go out and screw someone else so I do not have to constantly pester my wife."
—male, age 43

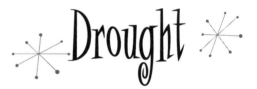

Drought

When an expert on TV claims that a sexless marriage is one in which you have sex once a week or less, some couples totally agree while most couples suspect honeymooners were polled to come up with that statistic. Gynecologists tell of some patients who complain of *only* wanting sex once a day and others who are fine with once a month. The most extreme drought we encountered was the case of a 72-year-old woman who, during 43 years of marriage, had only tried sex once or twice. Suffice it to say, what qualifies as a sex drought is unique to each individual, but the longer a drought lasts the tougher it is to remedy.

BEYOND THE DRY SPELL

A sex drought has less to do with a specific length of time than with an attitude that prevents couples from emotionally connecting. If your sexual encounters are constantly declining to the point where it is awkward for either of you to initiate sex, you are on a slippery slope. Whatever the root cause of the problem, it is complicated by the lack of communication or even denial that accompanies a drought. Often this is a reaction to the enormous social pressure to have a satisfying sex life and the near universal desire to feel normal. When we fear we are way different than most in any aspect of our private lives, we tend to clam up about it rather than advertise it.

Dr. Susan Bennett describes how sexual issues play a role with nearly all her patients. "I don't really specialize in the care of patients with sexual problems. Almost everyone has them, however, and I make it a part of my patients' primary care." Talking about sex is easy. Talking about not having sex is a whole different deal. Studies have shown that patients volunteer information about sexual problems 2 percent of the time, and are 12 times as likely to discuss sexual problems if the doctor initiates the inquiry. If your doctor talks to you about sex, or your lack thereof, consider yourself lucky, because talking can be the biggest hurdle.

THE ELEPHANT IN THE BEDROOM

A 42-year-old married woman who has gone over a year without sex and resents being told she should miss it asserts: "I still maintain not everyone wants to or should have to have it be such a priority. Some people, like me, just don't care about sex." Yet she is sad. Her husband is sad. They can't feel "normal" within their marriage because sex has become such an insurmountable issue. It is uncomfortable even watching TV together because the dialogue typically includes complaints from couples who haven't had sex in a week or a month. The topic of sex has become their proverbial elephant in the room that they deliberately detour but don't discuss. All the in-your-face sex just drives a bigger wedge between them, so somewhere along the line she and her husband chose not to deal with it, and life is going along fine. A lifetime of "fine," however, when it involves zero spark of intimacy, is uninspiring at best and a threat to your marriage at worst.

Healthy relationships are not all about the sex, but just as sex strengthens and supports the marital bond, a lack of it can readily erode it. Ask anyone from the call-in psychiatrist to the sexologist to the medical doctor and you'll hear the same thing. When a couple is not having any kind of sexual intimacy, it's usually a sign that something greater is amiss in the relationship. "Not having sex is a real barometer that something is wrong. People who don't have sex are not as happy, and they are more likely to leave the relationship," said Denise Donnelly, the Georgia State University sociologist. The subjects in her studies of involuntary celibacy in long-term relationships report multiple reactions, including feelings of sexual frustration, depression and rejection, problems with concentrating at work, and low self-esteem.

THE MARCH INTO THE DESERT

Certainly the stresses of career and family pose a challenge to anyone's sex drive. There are stages in life when both partners are so beaten and exhausted that drought is mutually perpetuated. Sexless relationships, however they are defined, typically evolve slowly and even unintentionally. Three days turn into four and then five. Then the woman gets her period and as soon as that clears up one of you is on a trip for work or gets sick or comes down with a festering cold sore and then you wake up one day and you're high and dry in a drought. Finding your way back to the well seems like an insurmountable chore.

"Because of our weekday schedules we always relied on our weekend mornings for sex, before the kids got up or even while they watched a video downstairs. When my daughter started playing hockey every weekend we lost those mornings, and it took a while to even figure out what happened, let alone find a new slot for 'our time.' By then we were out of sync." —female, age 45

There are multiple reasons why couples avoid sex, and drought can affect the least likely victims. One couple in the midst of a drought went to therapy and figured out they not only both wanted sex, but both wanted more adventurous sex. Each had been too shy to ask the other. Highly sexual people simply fail to prioritize it and can schedule sex out of their lives. The "perfect" couples who appear to have it all—money, looks, immaculate homes, brilliant children—are often smiling through drought, because something's always got to give, and sex is the one thing the community and the neighbors can't see. Hiding behind work and kids is not only socially acceptable, but also much easier than confronting the real work of maintaining a healthy marriage or healing a faltering one.

WHERE'S MY DRIVER?

Decreased sex is often is rooted in medical issues. We've already mentioned that 52 percent of males over age 40 (that's 30 million men) have erection difficulty and a contributing factor is emotional or stress related. Side effects from medication also can be the culprit. In a cruel bit of irony, some antidepressants and other widely used medications can impair libido or make it more difficult to achieve orgasm. Because it is widely assumed that "normal" men have an insatiable sex drive, men with low or no sex drive feel inadequate and abnormal, and rarely speak of their plight.

For women, menopause decreases sex-hormone levels, and insufficient vaginal lubrication can make intercourse painful and less appealing. Because the vagina gets stiff and fragile with disuse, lack of sex compounds lack of desire. According to Dr. Bennett in her lecture, *Sexual Physiology of Women,* "Decreased sexual desire or libido is the most common sexual complaint of women, with prevalence rates ranging from 10 percent to 51 percent in various studies. Aging, length of relationship, and loss of ovarian function correlate with lowered libido."

In women especially, low libido—technically called Hypoactive Sexual Desire Disorder (HSDD)—is a multi-faceted problem. Medical treatment until now has focused on the traditional, linear, male sexual response cycle of desire progressing through arousal, orgasm, and resolution. But female sexual response is different from that of males. Rosemary Basson, in her study *Female Sexual Response: The Role of Drugs in the Management of Sexual Dysfunction,* defines the "inherently biopsychosocial nature of women's sexual response cycle. If only the medical component is addressed, the chances of establishing benefit from pharmacologic intervention are slim." Translation—there is no pill to get women randy. When it comes to achieving orgasms, women progress along unpredictable paths that are greatly affected by numerous intimacy-based reasons that work along with their biology.

DENIAL IS NOT A RIVER

Once couples let their sex life unravel, it can be hard to find a reason to even want to get back. The justification behind the avoidance, especially when it involves a physical issue, can make it seem easier to let sex go rather than address the issues. At a certain point, like once a couple has chosen to sleep in separate bedrooms, it is even harder to find a reason to work back to a sex life.

> *"We haven't had sex in over a year, largely because my husband will not take care of himself. I work hard to take care of myself and when I see that he doesn't even make an effort it makes me bitter"*
> —female, age 43

Focusing on the negative aspects of ourselves intensifies the emotional aspect of sexual inactivity, until the problem becomes multi-layered and seemingly impossible to solve. One woman recalls from an extended drought: "He felt pathetic about his career, and I admit that lack of confidence made me less attracted to him, which in turn made him less confident."

Even when an effort to get professional help is made by one partner, the sources of guidance can make matters worse. Because sexual difficulties are highly charged topics, the patient/client is especially sensitive to any advice.

Bad advice can be especially damaging and squelch further efforts to get help, as it did for this woman looking to end years of drought:

"I actually tried to get help a few years ago from my male gynecologist. He gave me a prescription for some testosterone cream (that I was totally embarrassed about filling at our local pharmacy) and told me I'd better 'step up to the plate and fix the problem because my husband would find someone else to service him.' This is the advice women are getting, now, in the modern world. It's all about men being taken care of. It took me about a year to even admit that his comments were inappropriate."
—female, age 42

Some male therapists have even counseled women in physically abusive relationships to use sex to remedy the man's abusive behavior. This is frighteningly irresponsible and clearly out of bounds. It's important to remember that well-meaning and even well-informed medical professionals can set patients back if they don't consider the individual's unique perspective and circumstances.

ADRIFT IN THE DESERT

Sprinkle guilt and resentment into the mix and it's no wonder couples have a hard time hashing it out. Dr. Robyn Jacobs, a gynecologist and women's health practitioner in private practice, explains her theory on why couples have a hard time reconnecting after they drift. "When couples get on different wavelengths—for whatever reason—and feel detached, it can be difficult because men tend to need physical intimacy to reconnect emotionally. Women feel like they need emotional connection before they can have physical intimacy. Both partners may be trying to reconnect but resentful of the way the other is going about it." Many women fear that any form of intimacy will immediately trigger sex, and they want something in between. Meanwhile, the neglected man may either pull away sexually out of hurt or resentment, or jump too enthusiastically at the slightest invitation. Either reaction initiates an outward spiral of ever-increasing distance.

"If you don't have sex very often then when you do it is kind of loaded with expectations. It is like being lost in the desert without water for three days. If you do come upon a spring it is hard to sip . . . you just want to gulp."
—male, age 44

WHY GET OVER IT

In his review of Joan Sewell's book, *I'd Rather Eat Chocolate*, Dan Savage, sex columnist for *The Stranger*, a Seattle newspaper says, "Here is my advice to women with low libidos: You can have strict monogamy or you can have a low libido, ladies, but you can't have both. If monogamy is a priority, you're gonna have to put out, i.e., regular vaginal intercourse and the occasional tide-him-over hand job and/or blow job, cheerfully given. If all you wanna do is sit there and eat chocolate, you're gonna have to turn a blind eye to lap dances and mistresses . . ."

This is a no-holds-barred assessment of how the drive differential plays out in the worst-case scenario. Even among couples that deny their need for intimacy, deep down at least one of them craves a sexual relationship and no matter which partner that is, ultimately sexual healing can be good for both of you. One study claims women who have sex three times a week have fewer wrinkles. Sex is variously credited with creating physiological changes that relieve anxiety, mask pain, aid sleep, reduce stress, foster fitness, boost immune systems, stave off heart attacks, and possibly promote longevity. There is evidence that women who keep sexually active throughout their lives, have a better chance of maintaining a libido that supports a healthy body and relationship through menopause and beyond.

We don't need studies to tell us it's just plain good for your soul. One divorced woman who has recently resumed dating and having sex is keenly aware of the role sex plays in one's spirit:

"I feel like when I see older women now, I can tell which ones have maintained their sex lives through the years. They have vitality and a light in their eyes, which show a strong sense of self. I aspire to that. The ones who have not are on autopilot. They made their babies and went on to play out the wife role. When you do that you miss the part of you that keeps you young and playful."

RX FOR SEX: FINDING THE OASIS

Dr. Susan Bennett is unabashedly straightforward with her patients on the topic of drought. "When a woman comes to me and says she is not interested in sex I tell her, 'That's okay, that's normal.' And then I tell her, 'But you should have it once a week anyway.'" Bennett consistently sees lengthy sex droughts correspond not only to health problems but also to marital trouble. "People who have not had sex in a year—their marriages tend not to do well." She advises her patients to be willing to engage. "It doesn't have to be intercourse. Don't withhold sex because you're resentful, or give it because you just spent too much money on a wardrobe. We need to try to have sex out of compassion and to protect the nest and our family." Often the willingness to engage—to put the relationship ahead of our immediate desire, or lack thereof—is in itself healing.

"During any kind of emotional, physical, or sexual 'drought' the thing that brings me back from the edge of despair is regaining gratitude for why I fell in love with my wife and what I appreciate about our life together. Shifting my focus to the positive aspects of our relationship is very helpful." —male, age 44

Some say it's like riding a bike, but taking the analogy further, sex is more like a sport. It only gets better with training, and training takes discipline. Once you make the training part of your routine, it no longer takes mental energy and is suddenly less daunting.

WHAT DO *WE* KNOW?

Cindy: "One of the few times I talked to my Mom about drought she said, 'You just have to get yourself in the frame of mind. Once you get rolling, you never regret it. It is always worth getting yourself in the frame of mind.' She was right. So many of my friends have benefited from this perspective."

"I try to remind myself that I love my husband, he's a good father and husband, and that I owe it to him to try to get back in the mood and have fun."
—female, age 42

Edie: "Drought is a huge issue, especially because it is so hard to talk about. I hear many people contend that they simply don't want a sex life, when what they really don't want is to have to deal with having a bad or nonexistent sex life. The sex issue isn't like a stray cat that eventually goes away if you ignore it. It's more like Lyme Disease that moves in and drags you down. Sex itself doesn't have to be a big deal, but the stress and anxiety that *not* having sex puts on a couple is a major deal. It seems a bit backward but people need to take their sex lives seriously in order to lighten up and let it be an enjoyable part of their relationships."

BOTTOM LINE

Just do it—for yourself and for each other. Sex is good for the soul, mind, and body, for your relationship and for your family. Making sex a priority will actually keep it from dominating your relationship.

WHY YOU SHOULD CARE

Like it or not, sex is a key component to the vast majority of healthy long-term relationships and marriages. This is where you cash in all your chips and take some risks on new tricks. Plan away games, learn or relearn what turns each other on, do the little things that get you laid, and take care of your own needs so you can be available to help your partner. If the relationship is worth keeping, put it all on red, Vegas style.

WHAT YOU CAN DO

Men: You would probably rather sex your way back into a sex life, but ultimately that is not going to be enough to reestablish true intimacy. A simple communication breakdown can cause a deep rift and bridging it may take a leap of faith. Talk to your wife, or to a therapist, either alone or together. The one thing that drought survivors agree on is that it took work and communication to recover. If you routinely leave the decision making to your wife, don't assume she wants to drive the train in bed too. In fact, if you start in the bedroom you may discover that women like having some decisions made for them. Not her entrée or her friends, but certainly vacation plans, paint colors, writing holiday cards, and sex are open to your initiation.

Women: Don't use sex to manipulate—withholding it as a form of punishment, or offering it solely to preempt an enormous credit card bill. Do use sex to strengthen your bond. Take a page from organizational experts, personal trainers, and coaches: when approaching something that seems insurmountable—work on it consistently. Pick a reasonable goal for frequency and stick to it. You may not always hit your goal, but keep aiming for it and occasionally you may even surpass it. Get the possibility of having sex out there in the

> "I think we (women) are so good at the details of life that we detail the virility out of men. When we are yap yap yapping about perfectionism, it intimidates them into abdicating every decision to us. If you're always telling him what to do, why would he want to take over at night? If you want the guy to take charge, you have to give him the reins sometimes." —female, age 47

morning so you move through the day accomplishing the stuff you need to get done to make it to bed at a reasonable time. Unless you're a pro, it's tough to start sex past your bedtime. Commit to it in your head, and even if you're exhausted, remember that you won't regret it.

"My husband and I are madly in love with each other and are on a good, solid foundation, but I don't feel the need to 'test' our marriage. Do I think we could have a hot au pair in our house or spend long periods of time apart without either one of us having an affair? Yes, absolutely. Do I want to test that theory? Not really."
—female, age 33

"Fantasy is important. It allows both of us to feel more aroused and it allows me to feel that my wife is a little wild and crazy or even deviant. It is important after 19 years to feel like your partner is still a little wild. We like to tell each other different fantasies a lot of the time."
—male, age 44

Distraction and Fantasy

Monogamy is not always easy, largely because open communication is an ongoing challenge for most couples. Never is this more apparent than when trying to keep our lust, love, and thoughts focused exclusively on our life partners. When you are with someone for many years, at some point the grass beyond your picket fence inevitably looks greener. We've all been there, daydreaming about the sex scene in the romance novel, or gazing a bit too long at the tousled father at school pick-up or the yummy mummy at soccer practice, having a moment with the witty co-worker or the best friend's sympathetic wife, casually admiring the neighbor riding around on his lawn tractor or the yoga teacher doing her sun salutation. Distractions can crop up in familiar characters in your daily routine—the guy in the meat department, the florist, the FedEx guy, the barista—or from totally inaccessible yet persistent invaders like the old (and married) flame, the fabulous celebrity, the steamy athlete, or the alarmingly young hottie.

WHAT ARE YOU THINKING?

Distractions and fantasy fuel are everywhere, and are a fact of monogamous life. As time goes on and we become less fixated on pure looks there is a whole universe of men and women in all age groups who become attractive to us for different reasons. It could be the way a person is with kids, his or her sense of humor, the ability to have conversations or reciprocal interests. There is no age limit or physical standard required to stir distraction.

When we feel an illicit, unexpected spark it is often the freshness and uncomplicated nature of the person that ensnares our imagination. We don't see or have to deal with their personal peculiarities, pesky issues, annoying habits, odors, or agendas. Because we don't have to discuss who is going to make the kids' lunches, take out the garbage, or call the plumber, those people look all the more appealing. Sex with someone else is an arousing thought, but the reality ultimately leads back to smelly feet, hair in the drain, and the eternally disappearing toothpaste cap. In long-haul relationships, we are forced to see each other at our worst, while our attention fixates on our distractions at their best.

> "The grass is always greener on the other side of the fence—a pretty face, a young firm body . . . But those distractions are just that. You keep your focus on the bigger picture and why it is important."
> —male, age 43

To be sure, some people are simply not interested in or capable of monogamy, and get caught in the cultural expectation that funnels everyone toward marriage and kids. Marriage is arguably a social construct, and if there were more cultural acceptance for people not to get married there would likely be fewer adulterers and twisted fantasies getting worked out in shady Internet relationships. That said, if you're committed to the concept of marriage, you have to learn to deal with distraction with your pants on.

THE NEED-TO-KNOW BASIS

The key is to process distractions in a healthy, mutually acceptable way, tending to them before they take hold and unravel your relationship. Each couple has to deal with it separately or together in their own way, and it can be a source of humor or a dicey dance. Is it okay to go there if you need some help getting into the mood or to the endzone? Where do you draw the line between harmless fantasy and dangerous obsession? Do you talk about it with your partner and get it out there, or is it wiser to adhere to the "don't ask, don't tell" policy? Even among couples who accept the importance of having fantasies and share them on some level, it is key to respect each other by knowing at what level of detail to stop.

Our inclination is to avoid sharing or doing anything that will make our partner feel hurt or jealous. Denying or holding in thoughts may be effective for a while, but being open about distractions can keep them from gaining speed and generating their destructive force. Some couples openly acknowledge what young bucks refer to as the "Spank Bank," a place where they can access a memory or image to get them up and off so to speak. A middle-aged crew of friends uses the more family-friendly acronym JOMB—Jack-Off Memory Bank—and are quick to point out images that will or will not make it into the JOMB. Couples like this often acknowledge their fantasies in the spirit of humor and openness as a way to diffuse them. Letting fantasy in on some level, and allowing it some room to roam can keep the thought from dominating your brain space and make you less likely to act on it.

> *"If I don't tell my husband when I am distracted, it can gain a lot of power in my head. When we share distractions, rather than pretend they don't exist, we can move through them. By sharing I mean mentioning someone who is attractive. No need to share the extended thoughts of a distraction, but we both understand that a distraction means erotic thoughts about another person have moved through the mind."* —female, age 41

FANTASY TO THE RESCUE

Distractions and fantasy are not only inevitable but can even be a healthy way to incorporate creativity into your sex life. The romance novel industry thrives on our urge to fantasize, while cardboard boxes full of *Penthouse Forums* in basements everywhere attest to the same need. Although people equate fantasy with porn there is a real difference between using your imagination to summon images and simply clicking up a quick fix of Internet Porn. Using one's imagination engages a much more creative part of your brain and really, it's the thought that counts. Most people in solid, committed relationships can accept their partners' legitimate needs for distraction and fantasy. Some tolerate them, and others appreciate the added dimension they bring to their sexual experiences as a couple.

One mother explains how entertaining a distraction can rescue you from being trapped in the mommy zone where there is nothing sexual about your existence except for the living proof that you actually had sex. "A look from a hot stranger can make you feel desirous and desiring again.

ON THE LIGHTER SIDE OF FANTASY

"I have a crush on Matthew Fox's character, 'Jack' from Lost. I don't fantasize about being with Matthew Fox, but the crush is just enough of a chemical surge to make me feel like I'm not too old to be giddy."
—female, age 44

"I am not afraid to bring old boyfriends into my head to help me get through to the other side. C'mon, sometimes that is the only thing that will get me there." —female, age 37

"My wife encourages my fantasizing, in the hopes that it will keep me from begging her for sex." —male, age 37

"I was up front with my wife that my marathon training program involved going to the park, finding the nicest ass that was close to my pace, and fixing my gaze on it. My wife was just happy she didn't have to run in front of me for three hours." —male, age 41

"The threesome idea seems to be the coveted holy grail for men. There is something fundamentally there for guys thinking about two hot women getting it on and simultaneously wanting you. Some weird evolutionary shit built in there. Within a real relationship, I don't see how it could work. Too complex." —male, age 23

"I don't hide my sexual thinking or behaviors from my wife. I tell her when I see something in public that turns me on, but I am also quick to point out that I only use it as fuel for our bedroom. I also say that she really should be concerned when the spark goes out." —male, age 39

"For me it's all about the venue. I imagine I'm on an abandoned stretch of beach at night. It has to be a stranger because my husband hates the beach. I can't include him in the vision because my mind gets stuck on why he would even be there and that sort of kills my momentum."
—female, age 50

Feeling a little zing from somebody else reminded me I still had it in me." Another woman describes that feeling chemistry with someone else makes her feel sexier, which in turn increases her confidence and sex drive. "My husband ends up winning in the deal!" she says.

Maintaining distractions and updating the JOMB can be harmless and even revitalizing pursuits. Men and women say their fantasies are not al-

ON THE DARK SIDE OF FANTASY

Excessive fantasies, on the other hand, can be a red flag that one partner's needs are not being met.

"I don't think distractions should ever be articulated. Once I had a distraction that seemed harmless and private until he suggested acting on it. It was like an invitation. Does that mean I have to say something to my husband? If not, am I dishonest?" —female, age 43

"Though I know of other men who freely discuss how sexy other women are, to me that is a pretty major slap in the face to your wife." —male, age 40

"Not having meaningful intimacy or physical contact as part of a marriage can definitely be a deal breaker. If you are in it for the long haul and don't get these needs met at home, it is hard to get them met in some other way without really screwing up the marriage." —male, age 44

"I fantasize about sex with others when my wife is not interested in having sex with me. I believe in not having sex with others, but if a man's wife does not feel like having sex, how can you blame him for going elsewhere. Still, having sex elsewhere is a fantasy that I hope never becomes a reality." —male, age 43

ways about specific people but about venues, positions, and circumstances that they might not be comfortable with in real life. The unfamiliarity can add to the excitement. If it gets the sex drive rolling and all your partner has to do is jump on for the ride, it can be a good thing.

TAKING IT TOO FAR

Of course, some couples try to work the object of distraction into a ménage a trois or an "open" relationship. Those '70s-esque inspirations have a pretty low success factor, as jealousy tends to twist the main characters apart. If you have read the book this far, you probably aspire to maintain the one-on-one challenge rather than the prospect of an outsider or neighbor in your life or your bed. Although some couples claim that the tension created by entertaining the possibility of other partners is its own turn-on, others—even if they accept the reality of those fantasies—are either insulted or threatened by hearing the specifics of them. Acting on one's distractions, for the record, will be destructive to a relationship. Furthermore, the space between thought and action often includes a complicated gray area of fidelity.

WORKING THROUGH IT

When one partner does take fantasy too far, the only way back to trust is through extreme openness.

"In the beginning of our relationship, my husband and I were having difficulties with our life's direction—career, moving, and finding our shared interests in a new place. In this time of transition, I had fantasies about my old boy buddies, and I even had a moment of infidelity. Once everything was on the table, I was able to be honest about the fantasies, move forward with our family, and build a stronger foundation. Being truthful led to renewing our vows, which was about figuring out what we are about as a couple having experienced that. Because we were in a truthful place, having a baby together deepened our shared values. When we live in those values, every choice is the right choice. The road map changed with two kids, but our beliefs, goals, and actions are on the same page and life together is awesome. Bumps in the road don't faze us."
—female, age 38

Recreating limerance—which is spectacular because of its unpredictable capriciousness—is not realistic, but going off the reservation in our own minds can rekindle the flame. Fantasy need not be focused on a specific person. Some of it relies simply on variety that you may not have in your own routine. You can have fantasies and still be true to your heart.

"Sometimes allowing myself to indulge in a distraction inspires me to look at my husband with fresh eyes. One time we were at the beach, and I was deep in baby phase and not feeling the least bit sexual. I saw this guy coming out of the ocean and thought, 'Who is that hot guy?' Then he got closer and I realized it was my own husband. It was refreshing to know I was attracted to him in the way I was when we first met." —female, age 41

BEWARE THE FORBIDDEN FRUIT

You need to know when to draw the line. For instance the woman who said of her male friend, "He makes my vagina nervous," should not share a bottle of wine and watch *Wild Orchid* with him when her husband is out of town.

To understand the forbidden-fruit concept one need look no further than the fleeting Hollywood marriage, where one half of a hot couple is sent into isolation for six months with an equally hot co-star and unlimited cash. It is a wonder that any of them last.

WHAT DO *WE* KNOW?

Cindy: "I am such an unapologetic Tom Brady fan, that my husband feels lucky I don't utter the Lusty Big Gun's name in bed. I would never do that. I may bring him in as an appetizer, but I always send him back to the locker room when things get steamed up."

Edie: "Okay, I am a recovering Puritan, getting pretty bold at talking about sex but not quite there yet on sharing fantasies. Baby steps. That is the beauty of distraction and fantasy—it's your own private movie where you can make the scene, write the script, and, of course, cast the characters."

BOTTOM LINE

Book your trip to Fantasy Island. When used judiciously and with regard for our partners' likes, dislikes, and reactions, fantasy can be a healthy boost to your relationship.

> *"We're basically animals that eat, sleep, reproduce, and die. We're very intellectually advanced animals (or so we like to think) but at the end of the day, we're animals and we're kidding ourselves if we believe that rationality can overpower those animal instincts. If you put the forbidden fruit in front of someone for a long enough time eventually they'll get hungry and take a bite . . . even if they intellectually understand the hurt and pain it may cause."* —female, age 32

WHY YOU SHOULD CARE

By denying or being threatened that your long-term partner finds other people distracting, you risk creating or adding a wedge between you. By allowing each other that private indulgence you reinforce your mutual trust.

WHAT YOU CAN DO

Be open to cultivating fantasies but know each other's limits. Some believe the adage that, "It doesn't matter where you get your appetite as long as you eat at home." Others find that concept offensive. You need to know your partner and then engage your creativity to expand on fantasy from his or her comfort zone. While not everyone can find humor in it, accepting it will strengthen your relationship. Allow each other a place to go that's all your own, and be happy that it works.

♀ / ♂

My husband bought me this enormous vibrator—I am talking two feet long—for Valentine's Day as a joke. One morning he got up with the kids, and I decided to give the vibrator a spin. It sounded like I was firing up a leafblower." —female, age 43

"Women in porn are into sex, open, all orgasmic and shit. Watching porn makes you imagine what it would be like to satisfy a woman like that. Her openness is the turn on." —male, age 22

Toy Story: The Corner Porn Shop and Beyond

If you are looking for ideas to steam up your sex life with porn, costumes, and equipment, you won't find them in this book. There are shelves full of guides and detailed manuals in every bookstore, not to mention oodles of websites to help you work in extracurricular activities. Our mission is to guide you to the basic enjoyment of sex and orgasms. Whether or not you want to venture into the more erotic areas of the adventure zone, we think it's most important to master the mechanics and terrain of your own body and your partner's body as a first step. Sex, with your partner, preferably naked, is really all we're after.

IT'S HUGE!

That said, there has to be something to a $57 billion global industry whose revenues in the United States alone eclipse all the major-league sports franchises combined. Apparently you're not all just watching football and going to church on Sunday. In fact, as we interviewed people for this book, we started to feel like sexual Luddites, with nary a vibrator to show for all our sex talk. As one similarly tool-free friend maintains, "Those people just aren't good with their hands." To be fair, certain instruments do facilitate the hands-free access that some moral constitutions and comfort levels demand. In fact, vibrator use is so prevalent and heartily endorsed by both women and men, that it might be more rightfully classified as therapeutic than pornographic (see Taking Matters Into Your Own Hands).

Porn, per se, is not limited to the kinky toys and videos at "specialty" shops. Many couples admit to using some manner of erotica, either alone or together, as a helping hand to "doing what comes naturally." Beyond the obvious purpose of printed porn are subtler turn-ons men and women turn to for inspiration. One woman was surprised while moving to find a bunch of erotic novels that her husband had stashed away to get him in the mood, and legions of women merely pick up any passage about Jamie Fraser in the *Outlander* book series and break into a sweat. "My husband came home late from a boys' night smelling of beer and sausage. Normally, because he knows how that repulses me, he wouldn't have even tried for action. But I had been lustily reading *Outlander*. When he walked in the door I rounded on him like a tiger in heat." Watching a steamy sex scene in an otherwise legit movie can get a couple going, and we'll bet if Nielsen rated the bedroom antics after certain episodes of *Sex in the City,* there would be some seriously high scores. Couples go to a variety of sources for that little jolt that both relaxes them and gets the juices flowing, and certainly many of these do not qualify as porn.

> *"I don't feel that comfortable talking to anyone about porn, but my husband and I occasionally get a porn flick as a special thing to bring a little fun and heat into our sex life."*
> —female, age 43

PUNKY AND PIPPI'S WALK ON THE WILD SIDE

As the adult equivalents of Punky Brewster and Pippi Longstocking in our exposure to porn, we are not the ones to pass judgment on what is "normal." Certainly, our active imaginations include a healthy dose of fantasy, but the question we ask ourselves is: Where do you draw the line? To help answer that question, to educate our more modest readers who may be afraid of hidden cameras, and because we've always wondered what's in those shops people scurry by or scuttle into, we ventured straight across the line and explored some of Manhattan's spicier retail establishments. Here's a peek at what's out there, or in there.

The porn stores we visited were sort of like Target or Home Depot in the respect that they followed an industry-specific merchandising flow.

Gag gifts and cards in the front so the dabblers can make a quick, clean exit without penetrating too far for their purchases, and then products layered in ever-increasing naughtiness as you move to the back of the store. Racks of videos, as well as the "films" that pass as artistic, feature every combination of ethnicity, gender, and in some cases species (though not a single Swedish donkey film of lore). Books, magazines, and more gifts pull you in deeper. Even by Manhattan standards, we were blown away by the amount of gear that was packed into these small spaces. The corner delis have nothing on these places.

A PLACE FOR EVERYTHING

We were especially fixated by a common, back-room feature in most stores—a giant wall of vibrators in all varieties of colors, shapes, designs, and angles. Take note: laughing out loud—even at the vibrator with a lava lamp inside and the chocolate penis mold—is frowned upon in these places. Although the entire inventory is intended to bring more "fun" to one's sex life, shopping for this stuff feels like serious business. (For the record, we have heard of porn shops that are more like party stores with a cheery, carnival-like atmosphere. We just didn't find them.) More shocking to us even than the seemingly endless variety of vibrators were the frighteningly long extenders intended for simultaneous insertion in the anus. They look like a cactus you'd find in the Arizona desert, and about as comfy.

It's not like this form of backdoor pleasure is anything new, though it has gained more mainstream acceptance, or at least attention, in recent years. One man recalls his first introduction to the practice: "I was moving furniture for my father with some of his workers when I was 16. I hadn't had sex yet. One of the guys told me about a hooker he slept with in Vietnam. She had this scarf with knots on it. While they were having sex, she stuffed the scarf up his ass. When he was about to come, she yanked it out. He said it was the best feeling he ever had." Some people really do take fashion accessories to new levels and do, one hopes, frequent their drycleaners.

Modern anal beads are made from one piece of dishwasher-safe plastic with a ring on one end and descending sizes of balls spaced apart sort of like planets in the solar system, undoubtedly designed to eliminate embarrassing trips to the emergency room explaining how pearls got up one's ass.

BELLS, WHISTLES, AND BUGS

The stores offer up a solution for whatever itch needs scratching. Can't get no oral satisfaction? Try the Robosuck, the Hungry Bear, or the Tongue Tingler. No man good enough for you? Try the Sister Strap-on. Bored with housework? Pop in a few Ben Wah balls—they just sort of nest inside and ramble around up there while you vacuum or do your taxes. The variety and expense of the penis enhancement and hands-off male masturbation equipment indicates that plenty of guys think they need things like the Swell Guy Training Kit and the Facilitator. This is perplexing given the total absence of complaints we received about small penises and the stories we have heard from women reporting full-on multiple orgasms with guys whose penises are no bigger than their pinky (see Good in Bed myths). But then, the sheer size of the products we viewed on display—rubber fists the size of a Dustbuster and dildos that rival parking meters—seem designed to capitalize on the myths surrounding gear dimensions.

At an Upper East Side shop, marked on its brick exterior only by graffiti and a small sign, we took a long moment in the back room to focus on each type of gizmo, grouped by orifice and by degree of electronic enhancement, squinting at the wall as if that would make it easier to understand where all this gear was supposed to go.

The anal section and the vaginal section each had an astounding range of options, from the shockingly large fist to clit-flickers and remote-controlled "butterflies" and "ladybugs." A whole other crop of multi-taskers for simultaneous use in both orifices—beyond our comprehension—were in locked glass cases. Looking at one particularly aggressively shaped anal-stimulation contraption, one of us mused, "That doesn't look healthy."

"It's not!" a woman's raspy, smoker's voice interjected from behind the counter. "Of course men can fit much more up there than women." The storeowner then invited us over for a tour through the mother lode of the most popular vibrators, resting beneath the locked glass counter. She clearly favored the classics. "This right here, has been around for 30 years," she said, lightly touching a white, straight, modestly sized vibrator the size of a toothbrush case. "It's all you need."

RABBIT ALMIGHTY

We were dying to know about the Rabbit of *Sex in the City* fame, so I pointed to the thick pink shaft with lumps of rotating beads beneath its latex skin and vibrating "ears" sprouting in a curve from its base. The basic $92 Rabbit (among the growing rabbit family that includes the original Pearl Rabbit, Habit Rabbit, Queen Rabbit, Restless Rabbit, and elastomer Aqua Rabbit) features a rotating shaft with beads that move in circles within the G-spot zone two inches up, and vibrating extensions that externally stimulate the clitoris.

She turned on the Rabbit to let us feel it grind to life somewhat disturbingly. So many questions came to mind while holding the frisky "pet," chief among them: Where do you store it? How do you clean it? And how could a mildly self-conscious person buy it in public? One woman who got a Rabbit as a gift from friends did not love her new pet: "I ended up throwing it out. It felt so mechanical, and cheesy. Also I didn't know where I'd hide it. I can get myself off much better." The store owner admitted the Internet has hurt her business, but waved off the Internet's potential for her long-term demise. "I don't know how you can buy over the Internet. You can't feel the material and women really don't know how to estimate size."

Hmm. We've heard that before.

"They also can't tell how strong it is. These tiny women come in and want the most powerful thing out there. They're not strong enough!" she scoffed. "It also sets an unrealistic standard. No man could ever perform up to that."

We think that herein may be one of the dangers of sex toys and porn, in a subtler form than the Mardi Gras–like cover of the "gang bang" video at eye level. When introducing or glorifying the prospect of rotating or studded penises, there is the risk of setting the bar too high, or too low depending how you look at it.

WARP SPEED PORN

The old type of "static" porn is so outdated, that apparently, it's now quaint. With the advent of live-action Internet porn and interactive web cams, college kids claim they actually do keep *Playboy* around only for the articles. What they claim to get out of porn most is an attitude and willingness they can't easily find in real life. That distortion is precisely what *Time* magazine reported in 2004.* Among the claims made by the *Time* article were that porn is reshaping expectations about sex and body image, and altering how young people learn about sex. Men who are overexposed to porn can develop unrealistic expectations of women's looks and behavior, and have difficulty forming sustaining relationships and feeling satisfied.

Some young men are a bottomless pit for porn while others wonder why their peers like to watch something that is so incongruent with reality. "What is wrong with fantasizing about a hot couple having sex rather than jacking off to two midgets fucking a 400-pound woman?" says one 23-year-old male. "I once saw this porn site with two women sticking live eels in each other's assholes and eating them out. What the fuck is with that?"

---

* "The Porn Factor," *Time*, Pamela Paul, January 2004

THE TOO-MUCH-INFORMATION AGE

"My generation of men came of age in the era of Internet porn. Because of this easy access, porn influences the way guys view women, sex, love, and relationships. I would say it is one of the most important, yet least talked about, aspects of adolescent development. Guys don't see women getting pleasured . . . they see them getting pounded. They hear them scream, not moan. Expectations are turned on their head. People are trying to figure out the rise of sexual assault on college campuses. It's PORN (and alcohol and bad choices).

"Guys' expectations are way out of line with those of women, and again, I think porn is at fault. Most women I know don't watch porn. Most women I know want a monogamous partner. Most guys I know surf the Internet because it is convenient and accessible. Women in full, live video and audio having threesomes with gear, equipment, and wilder sex become required images to get off. In the end it is easier to sit in front of a computer screen than go through the rituals of 'sexual courtship.' All of that being said . . . nothing beats sex. So I don't know. Guys seem to love naked women lying comfortably in bed. I'm just not sure most of them really know what to do once they are there. Communication is key of course. I worry though that in this 'age of communication' we are actually losing our ability to communicate." —male, age 23

"Porn can become addicting if guys get too into it. The more you watch, the more you need of it to get aroused. It can skew guys' perpectives. We shift our expectations of sex to include deep throats, anal, dirty talk, toys, etc. I don't really know where to draw the line, but I know it is a slippery slope. Fortunately having a roommate limits my time on the web. There is a fine line each guy must tread so that he doesn't go too far over the edge with porn, though its convenience is tough to ignore. We get desires and urges at odd times and need to release when girlfriends are either not around or 'not in the mood.' Sometimes it is just easier and a lot more refreshing to use your imagination." —male, age 22

There is ample research that points to how porn leads to increased aggressiveness and sexual abuse, and leads men to objectify women. While for the casual user, porn in its various forms can spice up a couple's routine, the downside is that it can become a crutch, used as a quick-fix alternative to connecting to your partner and improving your sex life. Worse yet, it can actually distract from the task of trying to please your real-life partner. And, as our porn storeowner so clearly illustrated, it skews our expectations of everything sex related, from the size of gear or the intensity and duration of orgasms, to the visual image of what is really sexy.

All that said, porn is irresistible to some as an undemanding relief that is accessible, anonymous, and affordable. As one young man says, "Though it doesn't feel nearly as good as the real thing, porn with 'live audio' is a convenient source of arousal with no attachment and no entry fee. Sometimes this is just what guys are looking for." A more seasoned, married man points out that porn offers a behind-the-scenes upside: "It is incredibly demeaning to women in many ways, but I have a feeling that it keeps a lot of guys satisfied without having to seek other partners."

> *"My husband and I had sex until almost the day he died without ever using any of those things they sell in those shops. We were married 53 years."*
> —female, age 80

The real question is where the line of addiction or replacement lies? What is the difference between erotic and pornographic? Just a hint: If you worry about what might happen if your door was beaten down and your computer confiscated, then you might have a problem. If you are honestly comfortable about your relationship with porn, you may relate to this red-blooded male who says, "I think most people see porn as deviant, but I see it as more of a gradation of respectfulness to disrespectfulness. I like to watch porn but I really love to watch porn in which the characters involved seem to really be enjoying it."

WHAT DO WE KNOW?

Cindy: "I was amazed by the length and hooked ends of the anal gizmos in porn shops. Way back when I had only been having sex for about a year, an older, adventurous friend suggested I get myself a set of anal beads. She described how she and her boyfriend would stuff the whole string of them into her anus. Once she started to climax, he or she would pull them out, which would give her the most intense orgasm. When I expressed disgust, my friend felt sad for me in my vanilla realm but predicted in a smug, knowing way that when I reached my sexual peak in my mid-30s, I would see the light on anal beads. Here in the store, at age 41 and face to face with the new generation of anal beads—even though they looked far safer than my friend's string of plastic pearls—I was not even remotely tempted."

Edie: "When I lived in New York City, I walked by the neighborhood porn shop twice a day for three years. I never considered going inside. If I did look up at all I imagined inside a clientele who wore trench coats and fishnet stockings exclusively. When I finally did go into that store for research, I felt a familiar surge of hopeless inadequacy mixed with judgmental Puritanism. Such feelings were entirely justified by the front displays of raunchy gag gifts and nasty videos. But as we settled in for a long, cozy visit and watched the comings and goings of the customers, they looked a lot like the regular people in my neighborhood. None of them looked particularly relaxed, much less jolly, but it's New York for God's sake. Whether you're on the street, in the bakery, or in the office, everyone is just taking care of business."

WOMEN AND PORN

For the most part the women we have met who are into porn are resistant to fessing up about it and are especially reserved about procuring the tools of the trade. Be it renting a video meant only for the couple's enjoyment or facilitating the nearly mainstream use of vibrators, accessing any form of adult entertainment can be a humiliating ordeal. This 42-year-old single woman recalls the experience of replacing her faulty purple vibrator:

> *"I figured the shop where I bought my vibrator would not be very busy on a Saturday afternoon, and I could go in without being recognized. The front room was packed. When I went through 'the secret door' to the room with sex toys, videos, and bongs, I was shocked to see that it was also packed. When I tried to inconspicuously bring the vibrator up to the counter, the sales guy made this dramatic scene of opening the package and putting in the batteries. Meanwhile, the 'secret door' kept ding-dinging with a steady stream of customers while I turned bright red. The guy turns the vibrator on, but it doesn't work. He practically yells, 'This thing doesn't work, can you get another one to try out?' Cringing, I scuttled over to get another of the same model, having to face all these people before his second dramatic cock and reload. This time the vibrator works, and he proudly lofts it, in its full reverberating growl, and squawks, 'Now this baby is working!'"*

While the women in our research sampling who enjoy porn are largely silent, those who do talk about porn range from being offended to being unfazed, with very few embracing it as an erotic outlet. This may seem at odds with the reports that porn use among women is a fast-growing trend. But it confirms that women—if they are into it—are not entirely comfortable with it. Many women admit to seeing the benefits of porn if it is used as a bridge to a better sex life but not if it is used as a crutch or replacement.

With respect to their husband's use of porn, most women adhere to a don't-ask-don't-tell policy. Some are threatened and baffled by its role in the lives of men they know, some are disgusted by it, and others have a purely practical concern. This woman, who is all for her husband masturbating, nonetheless cautions him against watching porn: "It will only potentiate his need to have sex and he'll be all over me, which is pretty much hit or miss, mostly miss, and now we both have to deal with rejection and guilt (respectively)." Another woman doesn't care if he watches it, as long as he "is doing something useful like folding laundry at the same time."

> *"I went into a porn shop and left thinking, 'I don't need another dick in the house.'"*
> —female, age 40

In 1980, Candida Royalle, a former pornography actress, founded Femme Productions with the goal of directing and producing erotica more appealing to and respectful of women. Her couples-oriented productions are gaining popularity and inspiring more female interest in porn.

> *I was a regular internet porn user until I read* Female Chauvinist Pigs: Women and the Rise of Raunch Culture *by Ariel Levy. That book rattled my cage, and now I view porn in a different light."*
> —female, age 26

Even though we get it now, we are not running out to buy anal beads and raging rabbits anytime soon. We purchased a relatively modest flip-up penis pen as a hostess gift, and then were off, feeling pretty good about being Punky and Pippi. Anything that brings levity and mutual satisfaction seems okay by us.

Cindy: "I'm wondering how I have managed to have an active, fulfilling sex life for over 20 years with just two bodies together in bed and occasionally in some other place when we feel a bit frisky."

Edie: "Just hide the pen would you?"

BOTTOM LINE

People use porn to fill a range of needs, from facilitating arousal and fueling the fire, to speeding things up or feeding the most deviant fantasy. The thought of porn may gross you out, pique your interest, or turn you on. It's available, and if you have a high-speed Internet connection, it's practically unavoidable.

WHY YOU SHOULD CARE

Whether porn is a dangerous addiction or just the spice you need, it can have an influence on you and your partner. If either partner uses porn, or if you use it together, it's important to understand the role it plays in your relationship.

WHAT YOU CAN DO

What you do is your personal business. What you do with your partner is your personal business. What you do behind your partner's back will directly or indirectly affect your relationship.

"When I hear my friends say, 'My whole life is my children.' I cringe. My husband and I enjoyed each other most. We enjoyed our time with family but didn't require the kids to be part of our lives as they grew up. Fortunately, most of them were. We never had an intimacy drought and never gave up being a team. We had fun together from the day we met until the day he died."
—female, *age 80, married 53 years*

"Women need time to themselves—alone in the shower, in bed reading a book, a cup of coffee after everyone has left the house. I have learned to accept her space, but I am happier when invited in, happiest when she pulls my underwear off." —male, age 44, married 14 years

✳ Keeping It Fresh ✳

Older couples tend to smile and take a deep breath to consider the topic of how they've kept their marriages fresh through the years. Their gestures indicate it's a good ride but not an easy one and confirm that every couple has a unique set of challenges to face along the way.

We do, however, repeatedly hear about certain concepts that seem to be part of the success formula. Some of them—like maintaining and encouraging each other's separateness and tending to one's own needs—are conspicuously at odds with the storybook conception of "two becoming one." Other skills, like having a sense of humor, valuing communication and respect, and knowing how to roll with changes, may seem obvious but do not always come easily or naturally. Long-term relationships at every stage are a work in progress.

We know a couple, and we'll bet you know them too, because the vision of their perfect life together is an illusion that persists in nearly every community. For the sake of this discussion we will call them Ken and Barbie—strikingly attractive, funny, friendly, kind, and passionately in love. We can either torture ourselves with envy or choose to look more closely inside the perfect boxed set to see the same imperfections and challenges that we all must bear. Couples deal with their issues differently either by vigilantly covering them up (which will eventually blow) or by working very hard to keep the magic. It doesn't require date night every week, regular romantic escapes, sitters up the wazoo, constant personal grooming, and making every birthday and anniversary a big occasion. As unromantic as it sounds, long-haul sexual satisfaction is all about sustainability. Therefore what we really need to do is to define our likes and needs as a couple, then try our hardest to meet them.

Some couples manage to grow together so perfectly that they seem to be of one mind. We heard of a couple married 60 years who worked together for 40 of them, happily. Those couples may be our ideal but they are the exception. Time and again, we hear that supporting each other's sense of independence is a key component of many strong marriages. Maintaining and developing individual identities—be that through girls' and guys' trips, independent friendships, book clubs, classes, sports, or hobbies—energizes each partner, who then brings greater vitality and perspective to the relationship. We are certain that if men knew how much sex advice gets tossed around at book club, they would never again make light of that monthly ritual.

It's important to note that granting or allowing freedom is different from encouraging and supporting freedom. Someone who feels the need to negotiate or, worse, steal personal time is likely to spend some of that time processing guilt and resentment. When one gives the time freely, even happily, the space granted will more likely be used to appreciate all that's good in the relationship. Time apart also makes you look forward to the time you spend together. On the other hand, nothing says good sex so much as an away game together—a change of venue with no kids, pets, cooking, or laundry. Couples repeatedly tell us that time away together, particularly to somewhere that is a complete change from their regular life, allows them to see each other outside the stress and distractions of everyday life, and provides a refreshing boost to their sex lives.

What follows is advice for keeping it fresh from couples who have made it well past the seven-year itch.

LUST IN SPACE

"My husband's work meant that he traveled two weeks a month. We never had any of the intimacy problems I hear people talk about because I always looked forward to him coming home, and we never got enough of each other." —female, age 68

"I can tell you that a week away from work, kids, and family freshens the monogamous relationship." —male, age 45

"We have found things that each one likes in their own space and time. We each have obligations and leisure times that do not require the company of the other. We can shape things individually yet still have occasions to watch the outcomes together." —female, age 68

"I recently went away for the weekend to hang out with six of my college buddies. We didn't have any agenda except just being together. So many stories about our sex lives popped up. Hearing how others' sex lives are different or the same gives you perspective and motivation. It was great to have a physical break from my daily routine and be able to relax, focus on myself without family distracting me, and have space to think. Even shopping for new clothes put my sex drive back in gear and when I returned home I felt rejuvenated." —female, age 44

LAUGH IT OFF

"The ability to laugh at ourselves and with each other has been one of the key factors to staying together for 43 years." —male, age 61

"Have a sense of humor. You can't take yourself too seriously. When I get tied up in knots, it's when I have been very introspective." —female, age 60

"Have a sense of humor about your aging body, your aging mind, and your crabby pet peeves. Be able to laugh at yourself! Be able to be given a hard time or teased about your idiosyncrasies." —female, age 41

LOOK OUT FOR NUMBER ONE

"Care about yourself! When you feel good about yourself emotionally and physically you are more comfortable with your body and when you are more comfortable with your body, you become more physically attractive." —female, age 41

"There's no question that I'm a different person when I've had my run for the day, or when I sit down to a decent lunch." —female, age 38

"My husband was a dedicated couch potato until recently, he decided out of the blue to join an exercise program. It made me feel better about him and about us that he cared to make that change." —female, age 45

"I think staying active and fit is one big key. When we ride or hike together it tends to get the motors running in other respects as well. Several mountain tops have seen action after the ascent." —male, age 44

DATE NIGHT AND BEYOND

"I like the idea of trying to devote one night a week for dinner out— alone or with one other couple—and that night leads to intimacy later on. The man may think at least his wife is thinking about sex for a change, instead of knowing that she is worrying about the kids' science test or hockey game." —male, age 43

"We go out two nights a week 100 percent of the time. It's not fancy, sometimes we just get sandwiches, but it's the only time we can talk and decompress without stress or kids." —female, age 37

"I really don't enjoy going out to dinner often. I find myself staring across the table thinking of things to say and worrying about how much money we're paying for the dinner and the sitter. I would much rather go biking together or do something active." —female, age 41

AWAY GAMES

"The house and bedroom take on lots of other purposes and meanings over time—raising kids, getting rest, cleaning up, work, phone calls, and all the trappings of a hectic life. It loses its connotation of sexuality. We are big on getting away, to the bed and breakfast down the street or a trip thousands of miles away. I really think it helps any couple reconnect." —male, age 37

"Travel is especially bonding. You explore a new territory together and depend on each other for getting the best out of the trip. It brings us together even when we are frantic if one of us gets lost and relieved when we find each other again." —female, age 68

"There is the classic out-to-dinner date when I eat too much and don't get that excited for the end of the evening romance. Then there is the getaway weekend at some bed and breakfast. It is fun but boring at the same time. The best thing to happen to our marriage is an annual trip to Las Vegas. Vegas is Disneyland for adults—full of energy, beautiful people, good cocktails, and a feeling of eroticism that makes you drop your inhibitions. Plucking the two of us away from the daily grind and putting us together in some cosmopolitan hotel room with a killer martini bar at the bottom of the elevator is enough to recharge our sex life. Four days totally revitalizes our relationship and after that we look forward to hibernating again."
—female, age 36

"South Beach in Miami! Seeing so much skin, especially in the middle of winter, just makes us both feel sexy." —male, age 42

SPICING IT UP

"My number-one fail-safe method is something I call the 'Swedish exchange student.' I go to bed in some other room—the couch, the kid's bed, whatever. In the middle of the night I sneak into the 'girl's' room (my wife's) and pretend that I am sneaking into the Swedish exchange student's bed. BOOM—everyone is happy!!!"
—male, age 44

"For our 10th anniversary my gift to my husband was my first bikini wax . . . in the shape of a heart. It's great! It makes me feel sexier, and he loves it. I highly recommend it. The extra activity inspired us to put a lock on our bedroom door for the first time, which was another huge thing. I hadn't realized how distracted I was listening for kids. Now when we have sex I can totally focus." —female, age 44

"This is a very touchy subject, especially from the eager husband who wanted to experiment with new positions after 20 years and found himself out the door and regarded as some kind of pervert by his wife."
—male, age 44

"Night is when you are supposed to have sex. You're cozy, in bed. But nighttime is also when your stomach is full and you're dead tired. When you get older and the kids move out, you can have sex anytime you're both home. It's something to look forward to."
—female, age 60

"Try new things that get you to see your spouse in a new light. That includes things that you have always wanted to do, but haven't done, and would include trying new places for sex. Be game for spontaneous sex even though you're not in the mood. Sometimes this is the best sex in the end. It was unplanned, it was passionate, and it was fun!"
—female, age 43

GRATITUDE

"What I have found in a long-term monogamous relationship is that it is easy to focus on the few things that are not meeting my expectations instead of the many things that are fabulous. Once I fixate on the few 'sub-standard' aspects of our marriage, I am trapped and lose all gratitude." —male, age 44

"When your partner comes home, NOTICE! Make a fuss. Your children will learn to do the same without having to be told."
—female, age 71

"It sounds super sappy, but I think after 17 years of marriage, we are still really in love, and in the end that is probably the key. I am still a big PDA guy—holding hands, caressing, etc. I like a cuddle on the couch. My sister-in-law always jokes that with us it is 'Honeymoon all the time.' I don't disagree." —male, age 44

THE TRUTH BEHIND HAPPILY EVER AFTER

"Sex is part of the deal—not the whole thing but definitely part of it. It has to be good out of the bedroom to be good in the bedroom. I love her more today than when we were first married. It just gets better. The first 10 years were good but not great. She wasn't secure in herself in our relationship, and I was immature and overbearing. As our relationship went along she became more confident in who she was. Maintaining that separateness works for us. I have learned to cherish her good points and forget about all the rest."
—male, age 56

"The secret to a good sex life is low expectations. That's not as bad as it sounds. It allows room for long-term growth of each partner. The opposite of love is control. The marriage contract is not a conscious contract but the unconscious expectations of two people. I have mine. You have yours. You don't know the terms of the contract because you haven't explored it." —male, age 69

ALCOHOL

Alcohol sometimes has its place in relationships, especially in courtship. Many a couple might never have gotten together without first drowning their inhibitions or acting on liquid confidence. Some people depend on a cocktail or a glass of wine to relax them into the mood, or take the edge off a hectic day. Once you're past needing it to get in the sack, however, few people claim alcohol improves the quality of sex, and many attest to the benefits of sober sex. At the very least the amount of alcohol intake has to be somewhat balanced or else the whole package—the smell, the behavior, and the performance—is a total turn-off.

"Sex without alcohol is just better—crisper, sharper, and clearer. It's a lot like HDTV." —female, age 41

"One glass of wine gets me going but any more than that—or hard alcohol—pushes me into a zone where I can't feel and it takes forever to get aroused. I can't go there." —female, age 37

"When we go to a wedding with friends, we all go to our rooms and have 'wedding sex.' That's sex before the ceremony and before we all drink too much to have the sex we anticipated for the end of the evening." —female, age 34

"My wife is much more relaxed with a glass of wine or two, and less likely to be distracted by the pile of unfolded laundry and her book." —male, age 45

"Rather than conceal or fear the difficulty, we acknowledge, inspect, and laugh about it. Like most relationships, ours is riddled with imperfections. In our 16 years together hard work has paid off in all levels of our relationship—emotionally, physically, intellectually, and spiritually. Neither one of us believes we are soul mates—the only ones for each other—but our relationship deepens through open communication, honesty, and conscious gratitude about what we share." —female, age 41

"We did family, individual, and couples counseling at different times when appropriate. It is always a good idea to talk to an objective person as well as reflect on why you chose the person in the first place. Talk, talk, talk!" —female, age 60

MONOGAMY IF YOU MUST

Betty Dodson, our favorite pleasure advocate, asserts that long-term relationships are too much work. "Monogamy is a blight on the planet," she says, preferring the mores of polyamorous (multiple partners) society. Dodson may be radical in her view toward monogamy, but she brings up a valid issue when urging us to consider the changing challenges of monogamy. Expect that you will have physical and emotional changes, and be ready to change your game and your approach. At our request, Dodson offered her advice for those of us commited to the concept of monogamy:

- Incorporate masturbation freely, together and apart.
- Practice separateness as well as togetherness.
- Go on vacations together and apart.
- Mind your fantasies and cultivate new ones.
- Get your fill of titty bars and erotic male dancers.
- Get plenty of sex toys and play with them a lot.

"When it comes to sex, at this point we have realized that quality is better than quantity. It sure helps to know our libidos have matured together and at about the same pace."
—male, age 67

"The sagging body is of different beauty—not beautiful, but it gains supple softness, and we enjoy the touch." —female, age 68

"Listen to each other. Praise when appropriate. Look for the positive rather than the negative. If you look for the good, it is always there somewhere. When you live and love this way, good sex will follow."
—female, age 72

"Our marriage kept fresh because I didn't fall into the role of the obliging woman with the male in charge. I figured you have to have two bosses. It worked. My husband liked it when I gave it right back to him. Many men don't get it. Help around the house with chores, be part of the ongoing process of rearing children, work your butt off, stay close, cuddle, and whisper sweet nothings to your wife. It can have amazing results and it doesn't cost you a cent."
—female, age 80

"My wife and I made a deal. She promised me she wouldn't make a comment about my tractor and equipment purchases for three years if I stopped putting grub control on the lawn. The grass has gone to hell, but I have a new brush hog."
—male, age 72

BOTTOM LINE

Happily ever after is a process, not a destination. Monogamy is not for everyone. If it is the path you choose, head down it with open eyes, a positive attitude, an open heart, a good sense of humor, and a partner who shares all of the above.

WHY YOU SHOULD CARE

We all hope that "till death do us part" is a really long time, so it ought to be a good time as well.

WHAT YOU CAN DO

Read this book. Re-read section three. Dog-ear it and leave it on the bedside table. Talk about sex. Laugh about sex. Have sex.

WHAT DO *WE* KNOW?

Cindy: "Betty Dodson gave me some great advice that opened my mind. She reminded me that even though Bruce and I have a healthy, communicative, and active sex life now, I should be prepared for it to change over the years. She said it is important to keep communicating and adapting as we age and evolve. Who knows, maybe when I am 80, I will be swinging from a trapeze with a vibrator in one hand and Ben Wah balls in the other ready to steam it up. I'd better be careful, Bruce may hold me to that."

Edie: "There's nothing like writing a book about sex to shake up your relationships—with your parents and friends and especially your spouse. Certainly the research for my subsequent projects will not likely provide such a windfall of down-and-dirty relationship advice. It does bring up a cautionary note, however. When you're with each other for the long haul you sort of use up your moves in the first year or so. In light of that, it's a good idea to share the source of any great new sex information before trying it out with your partner. Some things—such as where you learned to do *that* are best not left to the imagination."

Conclusion

How does one write a book about sex? We found the more mundane and pressing quesion to be: where does one write a book about sex? It couldn't be at home because of Cindy's issues with clutter, not to mention her dial-up Internet connection, and Edie's fatal attraction to the laundry pile and the fridge. After one visit to the library we realized that was not an option either, as the culture of "shhhh" does not mesh with discussions that include the proper pronunciation of "clitoris" and the latest information gleaned from experts on marriage, sex, celibacy, porn, masturbation, and the like. Our ideal venue required a certain amount of ambient noise. Fortunately we discovered Dartmouth's Hopkins Center—the Hop for short—where, amidst strapping and nubile college students, two 40-something hausfraus are virtually invisible. In addition to a cafeteria, comfortable seating, and free wireless Internet, the Hop provided a steady flow of activity that kept us awake and provided an ongoing human study.

In the beginning our distractions were minimal—the occasional friend who wandered by, or the friendly maintenance man making a passing greeting. Gradually, the group of older men playing Go!, the museum volunteers, and the ladies who lunch, all inched closer to our table, perhaps hoping to catch errant bits of G-spot discussion. People squinted at our computer screens from across the room to see what was popping up that day. As time went on and our cover was blown, staffers, faculty, students, and other regulars checked in with questions and contributions. "How do you get people to talk to you about their sex lives?" people asked us when they first learned we were writing a book about sex. The real challenge is not how you get them to talk, but how you get them to stop.

Everyone either has something to say or wants to know what everyone else is saying. Be it group discussions in dorm rooms and living rooms, spirited repartee at social gatherings and restaurants, casual conversations in waiting rooms and on chairlifts, confessions on airplanes and road trips, or even unlikely revelations in the emergency room, nowhere is off limits for sex chat. To a willing ear, people volunteer information at any place, any time. All you need to do is open the door. This universal desire to engage in the discussion about sex reinforced our sense of purpose and guaranteed more material than we could ever present.

The most frequent initial reaction from women was: "I won't have much to contribute. I'm sort of boring." Men often needed reassurance that they were not betraying their partners by speaking to us. Once they understood the unvarnished and down-to-earth nature of our mission, the floodgates opened. Those with the most mainstream of sexual mores delivered some of the keenest and most helpful insights.

WHAT DO WE KNOW NOW?

Edie: "The Puritan Recovery Program is going swimmingly, as evidenced by a recent pull-down list of my latest-viewed documents in Microsoft Word. They included: sexless statistics; female ejaculation: fact or fiction; technology of orgasms; and strawberry rhubarb cobbler. This not only answers the question, 'Where is your mind young lady?' but also reveals the relative attention devoted to my domestic agenda. I went from not being able to say the word "vagina" to bantering about oral sex and the physiology of orgasms at cocktail parties. In fact, in the thick of it, I felt like my every conversation inevitably led to sex. The peak of this was when a discussion with my banker somehow swerved from my checking account to the concept of the sex account, and suddenly he was confessing the sex life lamentations he and his buddies shared. Whereas in the beginning I cringed at the sight of the book, *Guide to Getting It On,* lying face up anywhere in my zone, I am now unfazed by a full-size image of a purple rabbit on my computer screen and a copy of *I Heart Female Orgasms* at my side.

"So yes, I can talk about sex with the best of them, but that in itself has little redeeming value. The positive difference is getting past the edict handed down in childhood to avoid talking about anything 'unpleasant.' Not that sex is unpleasant, but the things that can get in the way of good sex are often unpleasant, or at least uncomfortable to talk about. Allowing people, including myself, to get over the big taboo about unpleasantness lets them unearth the bigger truths."

Cindy: "The rampant repression in our culture has inspired my ongoing informal research on people's sex lives for the last 20 years. My own defense against the force of the repression norm was to blow it open with humor and honesty, a core of my character, which ultimately led to my one-woman show. The overwhelming, positive response to the show was evident in both the audiences and the follow-up written responses, which led to this book. After a year of interviewing and reading about people's sex lives for this book, I am further convinced of this bottom line: Open communication is the only path to a healthy, balanced sex life.

"While this seems obvious and attainable, very few people are able or willing to take the steps needed to allow constructive communication to happen in their relationships. It is remarkable how many people struggle with similar issues in their sex lives, yet are convinced those issues are his or her unique burden. Feeling sexually inadequate at any level fuels shame in even the most emotionally solid, functioning people. Keeping one's family and job intact are necessarily the top priorities for individuals in long-term relationships; however, burying relationship and sexual difficulties doesn't diminish them. In fact it only increases their corrosive power and builds its own communication wedge.

"If the responses to my show rattled my awareness of the communication wedge that grows between couples, writing the book drove the concept into the ground with a stake. Humor helps dissolve the wedge. Even if it is a temporary phenomenon, once you are laughing about it you've already made a shift. Hope is always closer than we think."

CALL TO ACTION

The biggest lesson we learned from each other is that there is no best way to facilitate open communication. Whether you subscribe to Cindy's wrecking-ball style of laying it out there, or Edie's more measured approach of waiting for the right time and opportunity, everyone has the capacity to open up themselves and others. It is nothing revolutionary, but neither is it always a natural instinct. To be sure, our goal was not to be the keeper of so many intimate details, but we found that people's willingness to be open with us had a ripple effect in their own lives. Actions follow thoughts.

People reported back that our conversations—and even the concept of the book—inspired them to have more open communication with others, who in turn opened up by letting in a bit more light and encouraging their partners to do the same. Taking control of your mind, your body, and your life does not require major change. Rather it starts with subtle shifts, including an increased willingness and tendency to be open rather than closed about the snags that inevitably yank us off course. We hope this book, like Cindy's show, will be the catalyst to such progress.

We also hope this book inspires people to believe that sex is a legitimate priority. That does not mean that sex needs to consume an inordinate amount of your time, attention, and energy. On the contrary, by giving sex its due it will take up less of all those precious resources. Certainly the energy expended on resisting sex could power all the vibrators in New York. As for the resentment that brews amidst dysfunctional or unfulfilling sexual relationships—if you could bottle that you could annihilate smallpox, again. The purpose is not to force people to make sex their sole focus, but to acknowledge that sex is a vital aspect of long-term relationships. It is all too easy to take the intimacy and connection that accompanies sex for granted, to let it disappear through the cracks where, over time, the hidden pressure can silently create fissures that threaten a couple's foundation.

Because of our backgrounds, we tend to relate everything to sports: The benefits of team playing, goal setting, and training; the discipline gained through routine; the value of learning from your losses; the practice of capitalizing on strengths, while working on weaknesses within reason—these are excellent life lessons. Allow us one good sports analogy. In ski racing, as in most sports, if you don't look ahead, you are doomed to function in a totally reactionary way with changing terrain coming at you like a video game gone berserk. Forward focus keeps you on course, offers you some control over the situation ahead, and gives you the momentum to plow through the rough spots so you don't get stuck. Perfectionism is not only slow but also unattainable. It's not sutainable for the long haul.

And in conclusion, there is no conclusion. Your sex life—like the rest of your life—is a work in progress, and each of us can only hope that it keeps evolving.

ACKNOWLEDGMENTS

Our deep thanks go out to the following people:

The many participants who responded to our interminable, personal questions. Their honest answers confirmed the need for this message, led us down unexpected paths, and opened our minds. Without them we'd still just be chattering about a theory and some funny stories.

Alex and Susan Kahan of Nomad Press for helping us define and corral our vision and standing behind us the whole way. The Nomad team, for helping it all come together.

Joni B. Cole, who lit a fire under us and set the book in motion.

William W. Young, MD, Dartmouth Medical School, and Sarah Young, for that first fruitful discussion that reaffirmed the need for this book and sent us on the path to inspire healthy sex lives.

Laurie Foster (CNM, CPM, MS), for diving into hardcore territory with her fearless approach to women's health.

Joan Crane Barthold, MD, assistant professor of obstetrics and gynecology at Dartmouth Medical School, whose personal and professional perspectives are woven through every aspect of this book.

Betty Dodson, who blew our minds wide open with her extensive knowledge, wisdom, and conviction about women's pleasure.

Susan Bennett, MD, who supported this project and shared her personal and professional experiences. Her approach in both the classroom and clinic demonstrates how successfully one person can advance the awareness of sexual health.

Denise Donnelly, associate professor of sociology at Georgia State University, for sharing her observations and extensive research on those who aren't interested in finding the doorbell.

Robyn Jacobs, MD, for sharing professional knowledge from the trenches, so to speak.

Margaret Michniewicz, of *Vermont Woman*, for her edits and title for Mirth Control.

The Clean Sweep Reading Team for taking on everything from split infinitives to multiple orgasms: Rob Johnstone, Jason Lichtenstein, Pam Miles, and Michelle Sacerdote. To Jason, for the fine-tooth comb and global view.

To our readers for honest opinions, questions, and appropriate scoldings: Sarah Callaway, KJ Dell'Antonia, Josh Dooley, Ann Esselstyn, Jane Esselstyn, Charles Ganske, Rachel Gross, Caroline Levy, Lianne Moccia-Field, Patricia Parsons, Laurel Peak, Sarah Stewart Taylor, Michael Strong, and Daniel Tootoo.

—Cindy and Edie

My enormous gratitude goes out to all the following people:

Bruce and my children for grounding me, reminding me what matters, and keeping me on my toes.

My mother and late father, for supporting my renegade female program.

The original Panel of Wise Women, my sisters and sisters-in-law, who always find humor in bodily events and adventures.

My brothers, for openly processing their relationships at the dinner table, bringing great women into our family, and teaching me how to throw a ball the right way.

Nancy Pierce Williamson, my aunt, who always encouraged me to keep writing and inspired me to create, distribute, and sell my first newspaper.

My nieces and nephews, for being forces in the Pierce family soup and bringing each of their own spices to the recipe.

My nephew, Brooks Goff, and the Dartmouth class of 2006 football team members. Their respectful questions and openness launched this book idea.

The Coven of Lassies: Kristin Brown (The Maven), Jane Esselstyn, Elizabeth Keene, and Pennie Rand, for believing.

Rosi Dupre Littlefield, for inviting me on the Arc Angels ski trip, which led to the one-woman show and the book.

Kristi Graham (aka The Instigator), who insisted that the stories be shared publicly.

Jon Shea, for hours of kitchen sex chatter that challenged and expanded my perspective.

Magnum, who broadened my perspective of the male experience with honest and humorous reflections on all topics.

—Cindy

There are many people to whom I owe thanks, and most will be happy not to be acknowledged here. But I have to call some of them out:

Mom and Dad, for their lifelong encouragement and for being proud of everything I write. I *will* write that sports book someday.

My sisters, for always running offense while I slide through to the end zone. I couldn't have gotten far without them. They were right about a lot of things, including that the youngest one *can* get away with anything.

My brother, who took it upon himself to set the record straight about everything from Santa Claus to storks. I could have waited for some of that info, but he gave me a healthy sense of realism, and it all worked out.

Jean Hagan, for saying, "Why not write? It's what you like to do."

The ski team girls—teammates, roommates, and fierce competitors. I forgive them for leaving out some key chapters in the book of love, because they deliver an endless supply of camaraderie and support. For the record, Tori came through first on this one.

Deb Scranton, for giving me the contact high of chutzpah.

My many friends who let it all hang out, tolerated and answered my most prying questions, and trusted that those conversations would lead somewhere.

The Silent Majority, who took a chance and opened up to a fellow Puritan. Your insights will help many people to find a voice and use it.

—Edie

RESOURCES

Books

Chalker, Rebecca. *The Clitoral Truth*. New York: Seven Stories Press, 2000.

Dodson, Betty. *Orgasms for Two: The Joy of Partnersex*. New York: Harmony, 2002.

———. *Sex for One: The Joy of Selfloving*. New York: Three Rivers Press, 1996.

Hutcherson, Hilda. *What Your Mother Never Told You About Sex*. New York: Perigree Trade, 2003.

Joannides, Paul. *Guide To Getting It On*. Goofy Foot Press, 2004.

Lloyd, E. A. *The Case of the Female Orgasm: Bias in the Science of Evolution*. Cambridge: Harvard University Press, 2005.

Maurice, William L. *Sexual Medicine in Primary Care*. St. Louis: C. V. Mosby, 1999.

Miller, Marshall, and Dorian Solot. *I Heart Female Orgasm*. New York: Marlowe & Company, 2007.

Studies and Articles

Avis, N. E., X. Zhao, C. B. Johannes, M. Ory, S. Brockwell, and G. A. Greendale. "Correlates of sexual function among multi-ethnic middle-aged women: results from the Study of Women's Health Across the Nation (SWAN)." *Menopause* 12:385-98 (2005).

Basson, R. "Female Sexual Response: the role of drugs in the management of sexual dysfunction." *Obstetrics and Gynecology* (2001).

———. "Sexual Desire and Arousal Disorders in Women." *New England Journal of Medicine* 354:1497-1506 (2006).

Canning, D., J. M. Schobe, H. F. L. Meyer-Bahlberg, and P. G. Ransley. "Self-assessment of genital anatomy, sexual sensitivity and function in women: implications for genitoplasty." *BJU International* 94:589-94 (2004).

Chivers, M. L., G. Rieger, E. Latty, and J. M. Bailey. "A sex difference in the specificity of sexual arousal." *Psychological Science* 15:736-44 (2004).

DeVita-Raeburn, Elizabeth. "Lust for the Long Haul." *Psychology Today* (January/February 2006).

Didcock, Barry. "Sex on the Couch." *The Sunday Herald* (December 11, 2005).

Donnelly, Denise. "Sexually Inactive Marriages." *Journal of Sex Research.* Volume 30, number 2 (May 1993).

———. "Involuntary Celibacy." *Journal of Marriage and Family* (pending publication)

Feldman, H.A., I. Goldstein, D. G. Hatzichristou, R. J. Krane, and J. B. McKinlay. "Impotence and its medical and psychosocial correlates; results of the Massachusetts Male Aging Study." *Journal of Urology* 151:54-61 (1994).

Hunt, Carol. "For Me, a Man Who Can Find the Hoover as Well as the G-spot Is the Real Turn-on." *The Sunday Independent (Ireland)* (27 August 2006).

Leiblum, Sandra R., and Rachel Needle. "Female Ejaculation: Fact or Fiction." *Current Sexual Health Reports* (2006).

Marsiglio, William, and Denise Donnelly. "Sexual Relations in Later Life: A National Study of Married Persons" *Journal of Gerontology.* Volume 46, Number 6 (1991).

Mosher, William D., Anjani Chandra, and Jo Jones. "Sexual Behavior and Selected Health Measures: Men and Women 15-44 years of Age, United States, 2002." Hyattsville, Maryland: National Center for Health Statistics (2005).

Reistad-Long, Sarah. "The Science of Love." *Real Simple* (January 2007).

Scantling, Sandra. "Let's Talk About Sex." *OB/GYN News* (April 2003).

Seeber, Michael, and Carin Gorrell. "Sex and Your Psyche." *Psychology Today* (November/December 2001).

Song, Kyung M. "Trouble Looms When Couples Lose That Loving Feeling." *The Tallahasse Democrat* (July 22, 2003).

Tasker, Fred. "Sexual Healing Can Be Good for You, They Say." *The Toronto Star* (February 20, 2004).

Weeks, Gerald, and Jeffrey Winters. "Sex, What Problem?" *Psychology Today* (September/October 2002).